INVISIBLE DISABILITY

—— *Living With* ——
Macular Degeneration

CHRISTINE M. DONMOYER, PHD

Paperback ISBN 978-1-945169-81-6
eBook ISBN 978-1-945169-82-3

Published by
Orison Publishers, Inc.
PO Box 188, Grantham, PA 17027
www.OrisonPublishers.com

Table of Contents

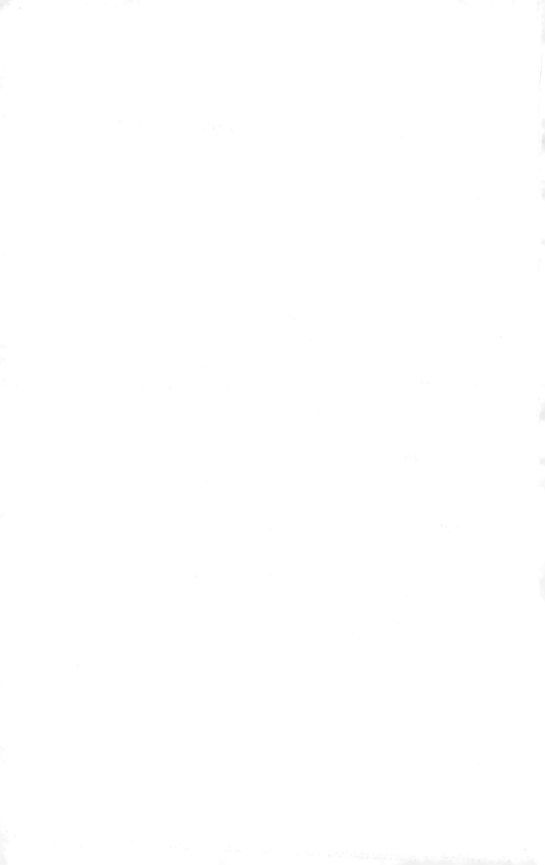

Preface

"You have the eyes of a 75-year-old." That was not the phrase that any 29-year-old wants to hear. Yet, it was true; my vision was as poor as that of people over 40 years older than I. In fact, some people in their 90s had better vision than I did.

It was the year 2000, and I was diagnosed with a form of macular degeneration that affects people under age 50. I am a researcher, so I wanted to learn more about the disease. I have spent many years on that quest. From previous partial lectures on vision in college and medical school physiology courses, my earlier knowledge about vision was minimal. Because of my curiosity and desire to understand my own vision disease, I altered my career plans.

Part of the original reason I went to graduate school to study physiology was to gain a deeper level of understanding of medical conditions. After my diagnosis, I had so many questions about my eye disease as well as about vision in general. That is probably why I chose to explore the complex biology of the eye.

I was in a unique situation when I was diagnosed. I was close to completing my degree in physiology and was contemplating the next step of my professional career. It was the perfect time for a change in topic. After defending my dissertation and earning my doctorate degree, I selected a postdoctoral fellowship to study vitamin A and its essential role in vision. Since that decision in 2001,

I have been extensively researching vision and the retina. I believe that the retina is the most interesting group of specialized cells in the entire body, but I might be biased!

So why did I write this book after becoming a vision science researcher? I had many questions about macular degeneration when I was first diagnosed, and it took me years to find the answers. This book is my way of putting the answers I found in one place.

This book also comes from my lived experience with macular degeneration. Understanding the biological science behind the disease helped me create a direction for my life with a chronic disease and disability. I believe that many people with vision disorders have a curiosity and a desire to learn more about what is happening to them. During an office visit, an eye doctor does not have much time to explain to a layperson exactly what is wrong, let alone how the eye normally works. Thus it is my intention, maybe even my purpose in life, to share the knowledge I have acquired.

As a vision researcher as well as a patient with a form of macular degeneration called Stargardt disease, I'm guessing I might be one of the only Stargardt patients who has performed vision research. It is my desire to share my knowledge of this field. Hopefully my experience also can be of benefit to other patients who would like to better understand their conditions. In addition to explaining the facts about macular degeneration in this book, I want to share my honest experience.

One early step of my writing project was to read other literature about macular degeneration. Had anyone else published something similar? I sought for a guide to macular degeneration, a resource that would explain what was happening to my eyes and what I could do to help my vision. Alas, my early searches yielded nothing. I thought that having some explanation of practical and scientific aspects of ophthalmology would have been useful when I was navigating this disease.

Although I found a few books about macular degeneration, what seemed to be missing were the emotional aspect of the disease and solutions to how to handle blindness. It was especially hard for me as an independent adult to lose the ability to read and drive. How did others deal with the lack of independence? In my search for resources, I realized that my experience offered a unique perspective on vision loss, both as a patient and a vision researcher. Thus I have shared my personal experiences.

I intentionally organized my topics in a non-chronological order, although some events obviously follow a timeline. I think of it as a journey where I learned many things along the way. Some events are distinct in my memory, and I have included the dates. As a reference for others, I think that it is useful to include my visual acuity as each change occurred.

The publishing team learned that a font called Maxular RX was designed specifically for those with macular degeneration, so choosing it was an easy decision. I also want to point out that I decided to minimize the use of italics, which are difficult to read, even in large print books. Instead of italics, when I wanted to highlight a word or phrase, I used boldface or quotation marks, which are more legible. However, italics are still used for book titles.

My goals for this work are to raise awareness about macular degeneration and to educate patients, family members and friends. I hope that this book offers to the reader the information and support that I was seeking and is a guide for people experiencing central vision loss. May it be helpful to you, your family members and your friends.

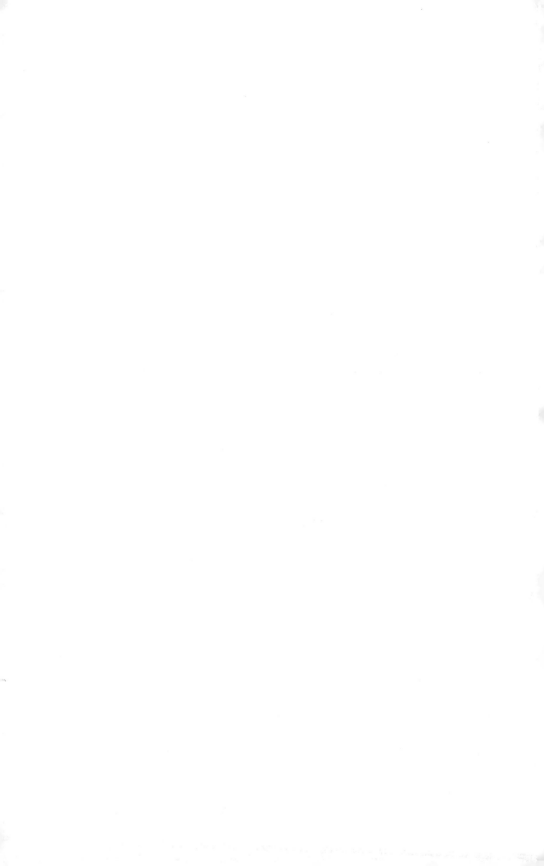

Chapter One
My Diagnosis Story

In 2000, I was a 27-year-old graduate student at Vanderbilt University, a private school in the great city of Nashville, Tennessee. It was my last year of a doctoral program, and I was summarizing four years of laboratory work to submit as a dissertation. In grad school, my intention was not to take the scientific community by storm but rather to obtain good scientific training. I expected to defend my dissertation a few months later, but as the saying goes, "Life is what happens while you're busy making other plans" (Saunders 1957).

A Brief Autobiography
Raised in the suburbs of Harrisburg in central Pennsylvania, I excelled at a young age in academics and music. I learned to play the piano at age eight and started cello lessons at age 10. I wanted to be a school bus driver when I grew up, a career decision that changed to being a teacher by second grade. My sister Corinne, 19 months younger, and I played outside in our neighborhood. We rode bicycles and swam in a neighbor's pool or in the community pool. Gymnastics, soccer, swimming and softball were my sports. My sister and I both have blue eyes and dark blond hair. I was an avid reader, tackling the entire Nancy Drew collection.

Our mother was a physical therapist, and our father was a switchman for the phone company; both parents intended for me to attend college. They encouraged me to pursue science with the goal of a career in the health professions. We were middle class Americans and traveled for one or two weeks for summer vacations. We were infrequent attendees of a local United Methodist Church, a mainstream Christian denomination.

By the time I was 10, I got prescription eyeglasses to correct myopia and mild astigmatism, which are both common conditions and relatively easy to correct. Myopia is nearsightedness, meaning that near objects appear clearer than objects at a distance. Astigmatism is blurry vision due to an abnormal curvature of the cornea at the front of the eye. To put it another way, my eyes were not correctly focusing light rays. I wore my glasses only to read the chalkboard in a classroom and to read music.

When I was 16, our parents divorced, and I got my driver's license, which allowed me to secure my first job. My sister and I worked at Hersheypark®, an amusement park with a chocolate theme. We tried to work the same schedule so we could carpool. After finishing high school, my sister joined the Army and was stationed in Colorado.

I entered college interested in pre-medicine and chose to major in biochemistry at Elizabethtown College in Pennsylvania, not far from my home city of Harrisburg. Continuing my high school activities, I played the cello with the Hershey Symphony Orchestra and joined intramural sports teams. I continued wearing glasses only for classes and for playing music. My roommates did not even know I wore eyeglasses, as I felt unattractive when I wore them.

After shadowing several physicians, I realized that tending to sick patients at 5:00 a.m. (the time for rounds at a hospital) did not appeal to me. Knowing I was in search of a career path, my college mentor, Dr. John Ranck, introduced me to graduate school and a Ph.D. degree. When I learned that many institutions waive tuition for students earning a doctorate in the natural sciences such as chemistry or biology, it seemed like a wonderful secret. I decided to go to graduate school in the biomedical sciences, where my goal was to help people by learning about causes of certain diseases. The information I learned could be used to develop treatments and cures. I was fortunate to not have any college debt, so financially this choice was not a huge sacrifice. Earning a Ph.D. would offer many career opportunities, and I was thrilled to be accepted at the prestigious institution of Vanderbilt University. I lived on a student stipend for six years, earning an annual salary of about $18,000.

Vision Status
At this point in my life, except for a few contact allergies, I was in nearly perfect health. At one of my annual eye exams in college, an optometrist recommended that I wear eyeglasses to drive. This was a sign of increasing myopia, a normal progression for many teenagers and young adults. A few years later, my vision worsened slightly. I realized that I should be wearing eyeglasses even when crossing the street because I could not see the Walk/Don't Walk sign clearly without them. At age 26, I switched to contact lenses. It was a helpful change, and I could see so much better. The world seemed to dramatically improve with contact lenses rather than glasses.

However, the optometrist also mentioned something peculiar about my vision; he thought that I had ocular histoplasmosis, a condition carried by starlings, which were common birds in the Ohio River Valley. Histoplasmosis begins with a fungus that infects the lungs and moves to the eye, and it can be treated with antifungal medication or by laser (Turbert 2020). Ocular histoplasmosis is a serious eye disease that is a leading cause of vision loss in Americans aged 20 to 40.

The optometrist drew this conclusion based on two observations. First, he saw lesions or pigment changes on my retina, and he was unable to correct the acuity of my right eye to 20/20. This number, 20/20, is considered normal visual acuity, which refers to how clearly a person can distinguish two objects that are a certain distance away from the viewer. The common way to assess acuity is by identifying the smallest line of print that can be read on a Snellen eye chart. An example of the Snellen eye chart is shown in **Figure 1**. I was not particularly concerned about having acuity of 20/25, and I did not believe that I had histoplasmosis. How could I have this condition? I was not a bird watcher and did not spend much time outdoors; my interaction with bird and bat droppings was nonexistent!

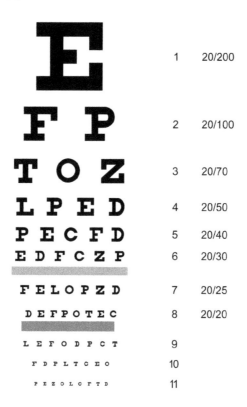

Figure 1: A representative Snellen eye chart

Returning to the Year 2000

By February of 2000, my sister was married and pregnant. She was having trouble seeing, especially when driving at night. Her doctor thought that she had some type of retinal disorder that could be tested after the baby was born. He asked that her immediate family members consult eye doctors to rule out certain inherited retinal problems. When my sister asked me to schedule such an appointment, I felt it was an unnecessary request. Clearly, I thought her vision problem was related to her pregnancy, as hormone levels change and can influence vision. I thought that she was being overly dramatic and that there was nothing wrong with my eyes.

During that winter, I had experienced headaches, particularly on Friday afternoons. Were they due to long weeks of work? Later, I recognized that the headaches were a direct result of my Friday morning caffeine intake. The headaches were prominent when I looked at the computer screen on Friday afternoons. They became so uncomfortable that my research advisor exchanged my small monitor for a larger one. At a suggestion from my sister, I changed the text color of some of my document files. My favorite colors were green text on a black background, but I also liked yellow text on a blue background. Perhaps the prior white background generated a lot of glare that bothered my eyes. These small color changes made a big difference in my getting my work done.

Doctor Visit #1

Despite believing that visiting an ophthalmologist was overkill, I scheduled an appointment at the end of March with J. Donald Gass, M.D., a well-known retina specialist at the Vanderbilt University Medical Center. Dr. Gass was an exceptional doctor, having spent most of his career at the Bascom Palmer Eye Institute in Miami, Florida. He had his own Wikipedia entry and was one of the "world's leading specialists on diseases of the retina." He wrote a book with images that describe retinal diseases, generally known as *Gass's Atlas*. This title seems like an homage to the medical textbook *Gray's Anatomy* (which, of course, was the inspiration for the TV show *Grey's Anatomy*). I could not have found a more effective doctor for this visit. Furthermore, he "pioneered the use of fluorescein angiography, a test that traces vegetable dye injected into blood vessels within the retina" (Pearce 2005).

The initial visit involved a number of tests before meeting the doctor. One of these tests, looking at an Amsler grid, was my moment of truth. I might even describe it as life-altering. **Figure 2** shows one example of an Amsler grid with black horizontal and vertical lines on a white background. When I stared at the Amsler grid that day, with each eye separately, I did not see the whole thing. Instead, I felt like I was looking through a donut hole. Please refer to **Figure 3**, which is a representation of what I saw. It resembled the bull's eye of a dartboard, in which there was a thin white circle near the center. I could see the grid inside and outside the circle, but the circle itself was missing or white. This was the first evidence that I had some type of vision problem beyond myopia and astigmatism. I did not "freak out"; I am not the type of person who overreacts to medical tests, but I hoped Dr. Gass could explain it.

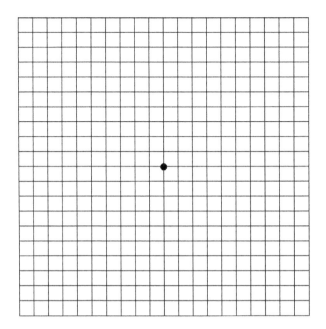

Figure 2: An Amsler grid

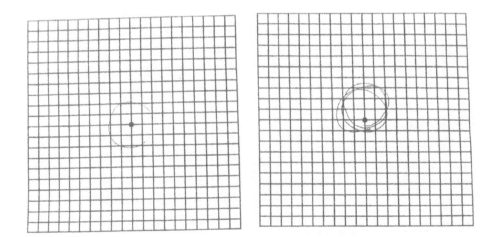

Figure 3: The Amsler grid from my perspective,
March 2000

   Dr. Gass applied dilating drops to my eyes, and I
waited 20 minutes for the drops to work. Pupil dilation allows the doctor to expand his view inside
the eye. He used a lighted device, an ophthalmo-

scope, to fully examine my retinas. Dr. Gass said that I might have a retinal disorder such as a retinal or macular dystrophy. The macula can be found at the center of the retina, and dystrophy simply means weakened or not functioning. At the conclusion of the exam, I agreed to return for a follow-up appointment in six weeks, during which time my parents visited ophthalmologists to determine if they had any retinal problems. Any problems identified during their examinations would suggest an inherited disorder. I was concerned by this possible diagnosis, but I was not panicked, since I knew very little about retinal diseases. As the adage goes, "Ignorance is bliss."

While still in Dr. Gass's waiting room, waiting for the dilation drops to wear off, the nurse spoke to me. Her message was that "it will be okay" and that I would probably not be totally blind. She should not have said anything at all and certainly nothing related to blindness. I had left the doctor's office with moderate concern, but her statement triggered panic; it was officially time for me to freak out. In hindsight, what she said was inappropriate and wrong. Total blindness was not what the doctor had said, so she was raising unnecessary alarms.

My thoughts included many questions: Would I go totally blind? How many years of vision did I have left? If I did become blind, what would I do with my life? The doctor had not mentioned anything about total vision loss. It did not occur to me then to lodge a formal complaint. However, a few months later I found out that the nurse was no longer employed at the Department of Ophthalmology, for reasons that I will never know.

Five Weeks of Waiting

What did I do in the time period between appointments? I did a lot of thinking and worrying. I thought about the power of denial. I had no idea that I had a vision problem until the evidence was right in front of me: the Amsler grid test. If not for my sister, it could have been years before I visited a retina doctor. The optometrist who prescribed my contact lenses hinted at histoplasmosis, which I dismissed. What if he had referred me to a retina specialist then? I was unaware that anything serious was around the corner. I took a short vacation to reflect on my life, which I describe in the next chapter.

I scoured the Internet searching for information about macular diseases—behavior that was unusual for me in the year 2000. I did not understand everything I read. I found little about retinal dystrophies other than that they could cause slow vision loss. There were websites describing various vision conditions, one of which discussed Stargardt disease. I remember reading a post from a Stargardt patient that described visual symptoms. What I read sounded much worse than a retinal dystrophy, which worried me even more.

Doctor Visit #2
My second appointment with Dr. Gass was on May 1, 2000. He gave me a short examination. I told him that my parents' examinations showed no signs of retinal problems. I had read about Stargardt disease on the Internet, and I wanted to make sure I did not have this condition. I asked for a fluorescein angiogram, which was, at the time, the only definitive test for Stargardt disease. In retrospect, this was a bold move for me, a 27-year-old, non-confrontational woman, demanding the doctor give me an expensive test. Of course, I had no idea how expensive the test was, nor what the patient did to complete the test. I thought it would be a simple test like the Amsler grid. Dr. Gass did not think I had the disease, but he ordered the test anyway.

A fluorescein angiogram test involves injecting a fluorescent green dye (fluorescein) into a vein. As the dye travels in the blood, a technician takes photographs of the retina. The photos show the dye in the retinal blood vessels. My eyes were super-dilated, and bright lights were essential to collect the photos. The first 10 minutes was intense because I was instructed to keep my eyes wide open and endure the lights, which was very uncomfortable. My natural response was to close my eyes to protect them, so it was a battle to follow the instructions as much as possible. An hour after the injection, the photo session ended, and my eyes felt tired. I wore sunglasses or whatever dark-tinted lenses the technician provided to me for the rest of the day.

"Christine, You've Got Classic Stargardt Disease"
The next day, May 2, I received a phone call in the laboratory at Vanderbilt. It was Dr. Gass, not his assistant, but the man himself. Although I was pleased that there were still physicians who made personal calls, the news he shared was not what I had hoped to hear. He told me, "Well, Christine, I looked at your fluorescein results, and you've got classic Stargardt disease." I did not drop the telephone or do anything dramatic. I asked meekly if the disease prognosis was the same, as if it might have changed overnight from our conversation the day before. I was grasping for straws and something hopeful.

The prognosis for a patient diagnosed with Stargardt disease is legal blindness, defined as best corrected visual acuity of 20/200, within five years after diagnosis. Little did I know then that this prognosis represents an average for Stargardt patients, with much variability. I asked if he thought my sister had the same diagnosis. He replied, "Almost definitely." She performed the fluorescein angiogram two months later after her daughter Rachel was born. The test confirmed Stargardt disease.

May 2nd, the day I learned of my diagnosis, became a memorable date, my personal D-Day. After the phone call, I remember crying that afternoon and talking with several co-workers, including my research mentor, Owen McGuinness. He reassured me that we would find a way to make this better. The afternoon was a blur; I did not get much work done. That night I was scheduled to attend my friend Carolynn's first organizational meeting for Mary Kay® Cosmetics; she had just become a new director. I went, and she asked the entire group to say a prayer for my uncertain health. I did not know all of the women at the meeting, and it meant a lot to me to be prayed for.

Post-diagnosis

I called several relatives after work, explaining what I knew. I told my sister, eight months pregnant with her daughter Rachel at the time, that she probably had Stargardt disease. She had already stopped driving because she felt unsafe. My mother and aunt came to my rescue and told the rest of my extended family my news. I was very emotional, and it was hard for me to explain my situation without crying.

Much to my relief, I learned that my support network in graduate school was strong. I was struggling with my diagnosis, and work was going poorly. One Saturday at work, a few weeks after diagnosis, I felt that my scientific career was over and considered quitting. Understanding that I was overwhelmed, my dissertation committee chair, David Wasserman, urged me not to quit that night. Instead, he advised me to sleep on it and decide the next day. He was right. I realized that I would regret quitting graduate school after so much effort. I did not quit, and we agreed that my focus should be on getting the degree. I would worry about a career direction later.

In June, Owen and I had a difficult conversation. He explained that at my current pace, I would not finish writing the seven chapters of my dissertation. This was a hard truth, so we devised a new work plan. Having a routine and an expectation every day helped me to focus on work. But when I was at home, I wallowed in self-pity. Nevertheless, by accomplishing the small daily goals, I finished the writing phase of my dissertation (174 pages!) and scheduled my oral defense for December. After many revisions, I submitted my dissertation to the Graduate School at Vanderbilt University and walked at Commencement 2001.

During this time of revisions, I investigated career paths. Someone had complimented me on how clearly I had explained my research at the dissertation defense. This led me to think that teaching and communicating science would be a good career choice.

One of the first things that my mother advised me to do after passing my dissertation was to travel, to "see the world" while I still had good vision. She suggested that I make a list of the national parks and visit the ones I was most interested in seeing. I was fortunate that my Uncle Chuck offered to pay for a trip to Europe, accompanying my cousin Tara, who had earned her medical degree when I was finishing graduate school. It was a great trip, and we explored six countries.

Medical Follow-up to Diagnosis

At another visit with Dr. Gass, I learned that he used my patient case for a Grand Rounds in Ophthalmology. Grand Rounds are regularly scheduled department meetings in which attending physicians, fellows and residents discuss patient cases.

I was pleased to have my case selected for discussion, and it was a treat to know that even Dr. Gass, an authority on retinal diseases, had initially not recognized my disease. My symptoms were mild, and I was diagnosed early in the disease process. There are more stories about my interactions with Dr. Gass in Chapter Four.

In the field of ophthalmology, there are many diseases with overlapping symptoms. In 2000, the field was still making connections between genetic cause and careful diagnostic criteria. Stargardt disease was one of those diseases that had quite recently been matched to a genetic cause.

Hindsight

I am so fortunate. I was lucky that my sister asked me to visit a retina specialist, even though I had no obvious symptoms. Who knows when I would have sought a specialist, if not for her insistence. I was lucky to have been Dr. Gass's patient and to have been diagnosed a relatively short time later. Some patients with vision disorders wait years for a correct diagnosis.

I was lucky to be living in Nashville and working at Vanderbilt University, as I was surrounded by a group of incredibly supportive family, friends and co-workers. My great-aunt and uncle, Rosemary and Jim Worley, had lived through many trying times, and they shared much of their knowledge and experience of disability and gratitude. I had a few close friends who listened to me and a bunch of supportive people from church.

I was lucky to have been 27 and not a child when I was diagnosed. As a general rule, the younger the age at which symptoms appear, the more severe the disease. Many Stargardt patients are diagnosed as children or teenagers, and their symptoms appear many years earlier in life than mine.

I am lucky to be living in the 21st century in the United States of America, which has the best eye care in the world. A treatment for Stargardt disease and macular degeneration is possible in my lifetime.

One of my students shared my story with his grandmother, an ultra-conservative Christian from the Midwest, and she calls this series of lucky circumstances "godincidents." I like this term.

Chapter Two
Coping with a Macular Degeneration Diagnosis

The nickname for this chapter is "The Roller Coaster of Feelings." This topic was the most personal and emotional for me, and I procrastinated many times before it became the right time to sit down and write the chapter. I am the type of person who does not like to dwell on her emotions.

Early Stages of Coping
Prior to my diagnosis of Stargardt disease, I accepted my myopia or nearsightedness, which was easily corrected with glasses or contact lenses. Being told that I would lose my vision in the future was an entirely different situation than my previous health problems. At the time of diagnosis and over the next year (2000-2001), I wrote in a personal journal. Re-reading that journal and reflecting upon that time was helpful to capturing my feelings, and I include some of them here.

Bargaining on the Beach
There was a period of five weeks between my first and second appointments with Dr. Gass, the retina specialist, and it was after the second exam that I received the diagnosis. That April, between the two appointments, one of my friends from a Bible study group invited me on a camping trip to

Destin, Florida. Such an invitation was not typical, and at virtually any other time I am sure I would have declined. Yet, given my heightened level of concern about my vision, I accepted the invitation. I knew I had a macular disorder but did not know any details about it, not even the name of the condition. Thinking it was a severe condition that might result in complete blindness, as the nurse had hinted, I was motivated to enjoy whatever vision I had left.

During that trip, I had an epiphany on the beach, a moment with God. I was sitting on a blanket with wind whipping in my face, fearful of the unknown, wondering if I would lose all of my vision. I wrote in my journal, "God loves me and will take care of me. Let Him carry the burden of my health. He has a plan for my life." I made a deal with God, a stage of grief known as bargaining. I promised God that if I did not lose all of my vision, I would be a faithful servant. I would carry out His work, whatever was asked of me.

Bargaining is not a new behavior. Max Lucado describes bargaining in his book, *You'll Get Through This* (2013). Many of us have a contractual agreement with God, such as "I pledge to be a good, decent person and in return God will do [insert request]." In my case, I was asking God to heal me or keep my disease from progressing.

Other Stages of Grief

Bargaining is one of the five stages of grief, which are clearly stated in Elisabeth Kübler-Ross's book, *On Death and Dying* (1969). She had a major impact on society, presenting a humanitarian resource for those facing loss of a loved one. She brought attention to the issues around death and the fear that many people experience about the end of life. Grief can apply to loss of a loved one, but it equally applies to loss of a relationship or a body part. In my case, it was the future loss of my vision. After my diagnosis in May, loss of vision seemed to be inevitable. I had been told that the disease would likely result in legal blindness, or government-defined disability, within five years.

The five stages of grief are denial, anger, bargaining, depression and acceptance. Stages can overlap, occur together or be skipped. The order of the stages is not critical, and many grievers do not experience these stages in any particular way. Some people remain stuck on one stage and never achieve or reach acceptance. I was no different; I went through all five stages out of order.

Denial
After my first visit to Dr. Gass, I was in denial about my vision disease. I pretended that I did not have a vision disease and that I would not experience blindness. Then I reminded myself of the results of the Amsler grid test, when I saw a bull's eye-shaped blind spot, and there was no denying that this was abnormal. I definitely had something wrong with both eyes. I continued in some state of denial, believing that scientists would find a cure for macular degeneration before my own disease progressed.

Anger and Depression
Learning about my vision disease was not a physiological shock; rather, it was an emotional earthquake. Soon after my diagnosis, I sought a counselor to make sense of my life and my future. She recommended a book about the grieving process written by Alla Renee Bozarth called *Life Is Goodbye, Life Is Hello* (1982). It is applicable to all types of grief, and one section relates to how a person's self-image may diminish with loss. "Some familiar part of me may have to die in order for me to grow into whatever new definitions or images I take on

in the normal course of life's changes" (Bozarth 1982, 27). Although I had survived an emotional breakup of a relationship, this was the first loss of a body part, or rather, a function. Grieving the loss of my eyesight took many years.

As mentioned earlier, I was angry and depressed after my diagnosis. Anger is usually not an emotion I dwell on for long, so that emotion did fade. Some days my emotions were overwhelming. I cried nearly every day for three months after my diagnosis. I stopped applying mascara because it began to irritate my eyes and stain my face. This may have been the saddest period of my life.

Social Isolation
Isolation and loneliness are two components of depression. Although my sister had been diagnosed at the same time, she lived over a thousand miles away, and we did not have a close relationship. I felt that I was the only one dealing with vision loss. Despite the fact that thousands of people are diagnosed with macular degeneration (MD) each year, I felt like no one else was facing this situation. Part of my isolation was due to not knowing anyone locally who had MD.

I was single, still fumbling into and out of romantic relationships. I was seeking a personal confidant, even though I had two close friends and my great-aunt. However, they had full lives, and I felt I could not demand too much from them.

Sadness dominated my life for a long time. You may wonder how long these feelings should last. The answer is that it depends on the individual. When John Hull, author of *Touching the Rock* (1990, 172), attended his first meeting with blind people, someone told him "that the time of adjustment toward loss of sight grew longer in direct proportion to your age." Essentially, the younger your age when you lose your sight, the sooner you accept it. Having structural defects in his lens and retina, Hull lost his vision in his 30s, eventually resulting in no light perception. He wrote in his book that it took four and a half years for his life to become bearable (Hull 1990, 150). I interpret this as his period of grieving until reaching acceptance.

I wish there had been a day when I woke up and thought, "Depression is over; time to move on with my life." However, that never happened, and it was a gradual process rather than a sudden realization. I spent a lot of time being depressed, dwelling on my fate. "O, woe is me!" In my journal, I wrote about being lonely and dependent, that "I want someone to save me, protect me, take care of me."

Victimhood and Fatalism

Stargardt disease is a form of macular degeneration. In the first article I read about age-related macular degeneration (AMD), Kals and Lauerman (2000, 78) referred to AMD patients as "victims." This description laid the seeds for how I thought about macular degeneration, establishing my initial identity as a victim of this disease. The age difference was irrelevant, as I merely had a younger version of AMD.

Blindness seemed like an enormous problem. I felt helpless, like there was nothing that could be done to improve my situation. It was the end of my world—or so I thought. What a defeatist attitude! In my journal entry from September 2011, I wrote that I was tired of being a victim. Many common situations seemed to be obstacles, and I gave up on tackling many of them. When I encountered a setback, like not being able to read a communication with Lyft after requesting a ride, one of my friends would tease me about my attitude of "Give up and die." It was my go-to motto, and it took effort to change that. Although these were reasonable feelings, I realized that they were preventing me from accomplishing my goals. I could not afford to remain in a self-pity mode.

Religious Thoughts

Early on, one of the thoughts I struggled with was, "Why me? Why would God allow this tragedy?" It occurred to me that one of the chapters in the Old Testament of the Bible, the Book of Job, addressed these same questions. My high school English teacher had chosen it as a reading assignment in my senior year. (Thank you, Mrs. Herigan.)

Job was a faithful man with a wonderfully blessed life; he had a large family and many possessions. Suddenly, his life changed, and he suffered three tragedies: his possessions were taken away, his ten children were killed, and his health deteriorated to where he was afflicted with boils on his skin. He did not curse God, but he did wallow in self-pity, essentially asking God, "Why me?" I did not curse God either, but I also pitied my circumstances. According to Carol Yoken, an expert on combined vision and hearing loss, in general people who have faith seem to cope with vision loss more easily than people who are not faith-based (1979).

There have been many friends and family who have prayed for my disease. One of my former students even found a Japanese object called an omamori, a form of protection, specifically an eye health prayer. I feel comforted when I think of all of the people who have prayed for me.

One of my well-meaning relatives told me, "With enough prayer, God can change the mutation and stop the disease." She meant that if I prayed enough, my eyes would be healed. I doubted this. Maybe my scientific training was stronger than my spiritual beliefs. I would be disappointed if I continually hoped for a miracle. Further, it would be false hope. It set up an odd counterargument of "If you do not have enough faith, you will not be healed." This made me wonder if there was something wrong with my spiritual beliefs. Finally, hoping for a miracle prevented me from accepting the disease. Instead, I needed to lean on God for strength.

Jennifer Rothschild (2002, 85) states,

We often think faith is a recipe for getting what we want from God. If that were true, it would mean that if I could just muster enough faith, I would no longer be blind. ... But faith is not meant to offer an escape from life's difficulties: its purpose is to give us strength to endure them.

The Grieving Process Repeated

Although I had no symptoms of macular degeneration in the early years after diagnosis, I subsequently went through many vision changes, which are noted in Chapter Five. After each major change, I repeated the stages of grief. Usually these time periods for the grieving process were shorter compared to the time of grief following the initial diagnosis.

About two years after my Stargardt disease diagnosis, I learned that one of the genetic markers for Stargardt disease had been identified from my blood sample. This was a strong indication that I had Stargardt disease, a figurative scientific nail in the coffin. I didn't blame my parents for passing the genetic mutations for this disease to my sister and me. After all, they passed a lot of positive characteristics, too, and you can't separate the good from the bad in the genetic lottery.

I began to accept my vision diagnosis. Although I accepted the fact that I had Stargardt disease, for several years I hoped and pretended that the disease would not progress. I resumed the stages of grief, starting with denial. Like Nicole Kear, I thought my "eye disease was part of my future, not my present" (2014, 9).

I had been instructed to schedule checkup exams every six months with a retina specialist to follow the progression of the disease. For years, I dreaded every visit to eye doctors, both optometrist and retina specialist. I wondered, "What if my vision is worse this time?" There was nothing that I could do about it, no matter the verdict.

More Vision Changes, More Coping

Reviewing what I wrote in my journals was informative. The first time I mentioned noticing a change in my vision was in the spring of 2003. Functionally, I could tell that I was not seeing as clearly as I had been. I cried about my vision change, and at the same time I was upset about losing an opportunity in my first academic job search. Then, in December 2005, my visual acuity was recorded as 20/50. My journal entries read that I "began to get more upset about vision," and I was "very sad about vision." I felt hopeless again, like I could not control my future. This is when I took the step to purchase a house, with the intention of making my commute to work less stressful.

In September of 2006 I wrote, "Who will want to marry me knowing that I am progressively losing my vision? … I have to keep telling myself this, my vision loss is merely a part of my life, it does NOT define my life. I am a fantastic person, no matter what my vision is." After many years of dating, I met the man who became my husband, Donald. My "woe is me" attitude of 2006 certainly would not have attracted him, and I had no idea what adventures lay ahead of me.

There have been many vision changes since then. Some of the changes were emotionally challenging, while others were tiny bumps in the road. The worst period was probably the time when I stopped driving, which is described in Chapter Eight.

Steps to Assist the Grieving Process

Many people have advised the following steps during grieving: taking time, counseling, having a sense of humor and laughter, talking to other patients, and reading books written by people in similar situations. I concur with these steps. I did all of those things, and here I describe the latter two items.

Talking to other patients

Soon after my diagnosis, I sought a support group for people dealing with vision loss. I wanted a face-to-face group. Most of what I found on the Internet did not appeal to me; however, I did find the Nashville chapter of The Foundation Fighting Blindness (FFB, www.fightingblindness.org). I contacted the vice president at the time, Peggy Mitchell, who was responsible for organizing social events and editing the newsletter. Peggy has Usher syndrome, a condition with both vision and hearing loss, and the vision problem is similar to retinitis pigmentosa (RP). She has become a close friend since that meeting. Co- presidents at the time were Laura Gammons and Susan Freeze (she has another form of Usher syndrome), a mother-daughter team.

Peggy arranged a lunch meeting between several chapter members and myself at a restaurant in July 2000. This was not exactly a support group, but they helped me to realize two important things. First, I was not alone in dealing with vision loss. Second, Stargardt disease was not the worst diagnosis I could have received; there are much worse vision conditions than macular degeneration. We shared that both macular degeneration and peripheral vision loss have symptoms that make daily life a challenge in different ways.

One opportunity that I passed up was joining a local blind organization. In Nashville, two groups were Prevent Blindness and the Tennessee Council for the Blind. But timing is important. Although I was seeking a support group, because my symptoms were so few, I was not ready for such a group.

It was disappointing that I did not meet many Stargardt patients in the early years after my diagnosis. I think that could have been very helpful for my psyche; however, I met a few people with different blinding diseases and life situations. Over the next three years I lived in New York and became involved in clubs and fundraising organizations related to vision and disability such as the Achilles Track Club, FFB and Fight for Sight. These groups were helpful in seeing the bigger picture of vision loss in society.

I attended my first VISIONS conference in 2013, sponsored by FFB. There were sessions for each inherited retinal disorder that they were working to cure. I met more Stargardt patients at this meeting than ever before, and all were highly functioning adults. I met a nurse, a salesperson, a student, a physical therapist and a film producer. If only I had met them sooner! Better late than never. I felt like I had found a group that I belonged to, a group of people who were succeeding in life despite a devastating vision disease.

Over the course of 20 years, I have met three other Stargardt patients who are college professors like me. One is now a retired ornithologist, another a developmental psychologist and a third is a physical chemist. I have learned some tricks of the trade from them, particularly how to manage certain work tasks with low vision.

Reading books
The only book I found written by a Stargardt patient was *No Finish Line* (2001) by Marla Runyan. Mar-

la told her story of earning an Olympic medal in long-distance running. Although this was an interesting story, it was not what I was seeking. There was no book that described what would happen to me as my macular degeneration progressed.

Many books have been written by people with vision problems. I focused on books written by patients with RP and Usher syndrome, which are inherited retinal conditions. I provide a list of recommended books and a brief description of each at the end of the chapter. One recommendation that I've already touched on came from a neuroscientist colleague: *Touching the Rock* (1990) by John Hull. He describes his experience of adapting to total blindness as an adult. I like this work very much, as it spoke to appreciating all the wonders of life. He explained the negative feelings of losing vision but has an overwhelmingly positive message.

Reality Check, or Gaining Perspective

Losing central vision is a big deal when it happens to you. However, there are many, many worse medical situations than vision loss. I believe that if I were restricted to a wheelchair or required to use a colostomy bag, I would struggle more than I have with the challenge of vision loss. Vision loss is not a tragedy, such as the loss of 343 New York City firefighters in the World Trade Center terrorist attacks on September 11, 2001. As Rothschild (2002, 79) points out, "Shifting our gaze to a bigger problem will put our own situation in perspective."

My friend Hilary Ann was a medical student when I was diagnosed. She gave me an inspirational book titled *Postcards for People Who Hurt* (1995) by Claire Cloninger, which had daily, one-page devotional messages. Hilary Ann had overcome many physical and professional obstacles, such as surviving a pituitary tumor and training for Ironman competitions. Knowing her story was helpful because my problems seemed smaller.

Someone else will always have it worse than us. For me, my physical challenge is my eyes; for others, the challenge may be cognitive or loss of limbs. Sometimes I need to remind myself that Stargardt disease is not fatal. My obituary will not read "cause of death, Stargardt disease." Instead, my obituary will cover what I did during my life. I can walk, talk, think and remember. My vision problem barely affects my mobility.

Although vision loss is not a life-ending situation, it certainly is life-altering. I was not able to anticipate all of the ways that vision loss would alter my life. I began to re-think what I wanted in life; it is doubtful that would have happened without the diagnosis. However, it was a relief to learn that the prognosis for Stargardt disease varies widely among patients. My sister's vision deteriorated rapidly, leading to a change in job responsibilities and then having to leave her position and sign up for disability payments. I wondered if this would be my path as well.

Advice

My advice to people facing macular degeneration or other vision loss is to collect as much information as possible about the condition, including potential treatments. Knowledge leads to informed decisions. Fear of the known is less scary than fear of the unknown. Think positively and approach life with a sense of humor.

In hindsight, I am fortunate to have been diagnosed at Vanderbilt, surrounded by friends and family. Finishing my doctorate degree was an appropriate time to consider a career change; it was the best place for me to be, among close friends and family.

Positives of Vision Loss

There are some positive things about a macular degeneration diagnosis. Driving fast is no longer a priority. In fact, I would never again be the designated driver that others would trust to drive them home after drinking alcohol. So, I embraced the opportunity. Now I could drink freely after having arranged transportation!

I spend less time worrying about my physical appearance. Blemishes and wrinkles are less noticeable. People's faces appear beautiful to me, better than when I could see with 20/30 acuity. I appreciate my friends and family more deeply. I have empathy for others experiencing illness.

Motivational Thoughts and Quotations

"We get 15 minutes in Pity City, but we can't live there." Author Unknown

"I had no shoes and complained until I met a person who had no feet." Persian proverb

"Success is liking yourself, liking what you do, and liking how you do it." Maya Angelou

"Non nobis solum nati sumus. (We are not born for ourselves alone.)" Cicero

"People are like stained-glass windows. They sparkle and shine when the sun is out, but when the darkness sets in, their true beauty is revealed only if there is a light from within." Elisabeth Kübler-Ross

Wisdom from Other Blind Folks

At another VISIONS conference sponsored by FFB, I heard an inspirational quote from Jim Platzer of Fort Wayne, Indiana: "Think outside our perceived limitations."

John Hull (1990, 78) wrote, "There are some situations in life when you have to carry out a protracted but dignified warfare against despair and not allow yourself to be made the emotional slave of those who offer false hopes."

"Self-pity is our worst enemy and if we yield to it, we can never do anything wise in this world," said Helen Keller.

My Final Three Nuggets of Wisdom

1. Do not take yourself too seriously. Break the tendencies of perfectionism.

Mistakes happen, and more mistakes happen when you can't see fully. One morning I put lentils in my yogurt because the lentil bag was remarkably similar to the granola bag. I was able to laugh at myself about it.

2. Do not believe the negative things that others say about you. They are belittlers, and they do not know all that you are capable of doing.

There is a stigma to vision loss, and well-meaning people can fall into this trap. You are the best person to assess what you can do. Live life to the fullest. Don't let anyone tell you who you can or cannot be.

3. Be comfortable in your own skin.

Losing vision is an adjustment. Accept what you can and cannot do, and others will follow suit.

Recommended Readings

The following books are true stories about life without vision or the experience of losing vision from particular vision diseases, in annotated bibliography format.

Alexander, Rebecca. *Not Fade Away: A Memoir of Senses Lost and Found.* Mexico: Thorndike Press, 2014.

Rebecca explains Usher syndrome (vision and hearing loss) and getting a cochlear implant.

Grunwald, Henry. *Twilight: Losing Sight, Gaining Insight*. New York: Alfred A. Knopf, 1999.

Dealing with wet AMD, Grunwald describes the state-of-the-art low vision devices at the end of the 20th century.

Hingson, Michael. *Thunder Dog*. Nashville: Thomas Nelson, 2011.

Blind from birth due to retinopathy of prematurity, Michael describes how his guide dog Roselle helped him exit the World Trade Center from the 78th floor on that fateful day of September 11, 2001.

Hull, John M. *Touching the Rock: An Experience of Blindness*. New York: Pantheon, 1990.

This is a descriptive account of losing vision as an adult and adapting to a new life.

Kear, Nicole C. *Now I See You*. Blackstone Audio, 2014.

Nicole was diagnosed with retinitis pigmentosa at age 19 and discusses blindness and motherhood. Some cursing.

Knighton, Ryan. *Cockeyed: A Memoir*. New York: Public Affairs, 2006.

Ryan has an amusing and quirky life with retinitis pigmentosa.

Knipfel, Jim. *Slack Jaw*. New York: Penguin Putnam, 1999.

Jim views life with retinitis pigmentosa with an appreciation of darkness and the absurd. Some cursing.

Mink, Deborah A. *Adapting to Vision Challenges—Together*. Self-published, 2020.

This recent publication describes the experiences of a loving couple when one partner loses vision, with tips on daily living.

Rothschild, Jennifer. *Lessons I Learned in the Dark: Steps to Walking by Faith, Not by Sight*. Colorado Springs: Multnomah Books, 2002.

Jennifer has a Christian message while dealing with retinitis pigmentosa.

Runyan, Marla. *No Finish Line: My Life as I See It.* New York: G.P. Putnam Sons, 2001.

Diagnosed as a child with Stargardt disease, Marla recounts her training as a distance runner and winning an Olympic medal.

Chapter Three
History of Vision Theory and Biology of the Retina

This chapter contains what I consider to be the basic scientific information about human vision and some historical highlights of how this theory developed. It is not intended to explain all of the intricacies of human vision.

What Is Vision?

Vision, or sight, is a sense that many species of animals, including humans, use to detect signals in their environment. According to fossil records, some animals have lost the ability to see, such as cave-dwelling fish, whereas other animals have improved their sight by various modifications. The most basic level of sight is light perception, which is the ability to detect light in the external environment. This is useful for setting a sleep cycle or circadian rhythm, which organizes body processes for certain times of day or night. Regardless of the environmental light conditions, many animals wake and perform daily activities at the same time every day. Even non-animals like algae have a light-detecting spot used for circadian rhythms and photosynthesis, allowing them to use the sun for energy. As they move toward the light, they are able to use energy more efficiently and grow. In dim or dark lighting conditions, they store energy and rest.

If the first level of vision is detecting light versus dark, the next levels of vision are detecting motion and perceiving objects. Distinguishing an object requires spatial resolution, meaning sharpness and clarity, or the ability to detect fine detail. To accomplish this, animals evolved two basic variations of eye design, or optical systems, known as the compound eye and the camera eye, as shown in **Figure 4**. Animals like arthropods (crabs, cuttlefish and spiders) have compound eyes containing arrays of internal lenses that send light to a few photoreceptor cells within their eyes. This style offers a wide field of view and moderate spatial resolution that is effective for small animals to see their environment, eat and avoid predators (Lamb 2001, 66). The fantastically colored mantis shrimp has compound eyes that offer moderate spatial resolution. However, it possesses six types of photoreceptors, or light-detecting cells, that give it enhanced sensation. The photoreceptors (12 in total) allow the mantis shrimp to detect ultraviolet (UV) light. It should be clear now how complicated the process of sight and vision can be with so many different variables at play.

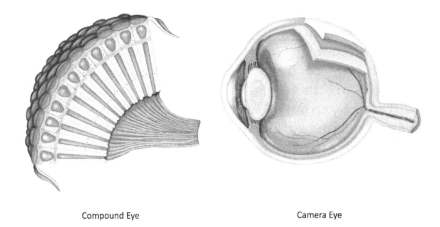

Compound Eye   Camera Eye

Figure 4: A visual comparison of eye types with compound (dragonfly) and camera-style (human). Drawing by Bryce Olson

Mammals, including humans, have a camera eye with a single lens that focuses light rays from the outside world onto many photoreceptors. This style is more effective for larger animals. There are two types of photoreceptors preset in the eye: rods and cones. Cones operate in conditions of bright light and enable detailed, color vision. Rods operate in dim light conditions and enable differentiation between light and dark. Rods also enable the detection of motion, especially in the peripheral field of vision. Nearly all mammals are rod-dominant, whereas birds are cone-dominant, indicating which photoreceptor type is more abundant. Humans have excellent color vision, but other animal classes—fish, reptiles and birds—have even more effective color vision since they have a greater number of cone photoreceptors (Kolb 2003, 28). Birds of prey, such as hawks, have advanced focusing abilities and higher photoreceptor density, allowing for very high acuity or extremely detailed vision. These specialized adaptations allow them to see much farther than humans (Fitzgerald 2018, 93). Altogether, our animal kingdom has diverse vision capabilities, depending on the number and organization of photoreceptors in the eye.

Basic Eye Anatomy
The three basic parts of the eye are the cornea, lens and retina, as shown in **Figure 5**. As light enters the eye, the cornea and lens bend the rays, passing them through the vitreous humor. The vitreous humor is a watery mixture with the consistency of jelly that supports the spherical shape of the eye. The rays are aimed toward the back of the eye onto the retina. The retina contains the eye's light-sensitive neurons known as photoreceptors. Neurons are structures that receive signals and send signals to other neurons. They use an enormous amount of cellular energy in

the form of adenosine triphosphatte (ATP). Once a photoreceptor is stimulated by light, it sends a signal to neighboring neurons. This signal is then transmitted to the optic nerve, which passes it on to the occipital lobe. The occipital lobe is the part of the brain responsible for the processing and perception of vision.

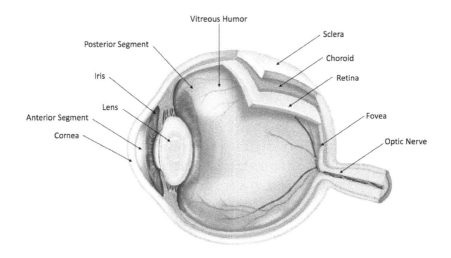

Figure 5: Basic human eye anatomy of cornea, lens, vitreous humor and retina. Drawing by Bryce Olson

The retina is an extension of the brain. Although I often emphasize to students how important the retina is, in historical terms, many of the early philosopher-scientists ignored it, with noted exceptions being Galen and Hunayn. In the ancient world, the retina was the Rodney Dangerfield of the eye: it "got no respect."

History of Vision Theory
How did previous generations think vision occurred?

Virtually none of my post-doctoral training in vision research mentioned a history of the field. Learning about historical perspectives is not a "hot topic" for scientists, and frequently the people who study it are historians of science. That being said, I enjoyed reading A. Mark Smith's book, *From Sight to Light* (2015). This scholarly work is a detailed history of the field of optics from ancient to modern times. How the ancient philosophers explained vision was interesting to me, as well as how this perspective changed into what I was taught in the 21st century.

Smith takes the reader on a journey through mathematics, specifically ray geometry, to explain properties of mirrors, such as reflection. He addresses the behavior of light in the different media of air and water. He describes how the natural philosophers conceived sight, drawing from a wide range of writings including ancient Greeks (Plato, Aristotle, Euclid), Romans (Ptolemy, Galen) and Arabs (Alhacen, Avicenna). Alhacen wrote that optic nerves "provide conduits for the cerebral spirit that renders the lens visually sensitive" (Smith 2015, 187-190). Although later scientists would demonstrate that he was incorrect, as the optic nerve is actually used to communicate signals to the brain, at least he understood that the lens and optic nerves play roles in vision.

The visual theory took these writers and many other contributors centuries to formulate. By the year 1150, the general theory of vision entailed the following: "The visual act begins with the emission of luminous flux from the center of the eye along straight lines within a cone of radiation" (Smith 2015, 234). Luminous flux originates in the brain's "innate spirit" and is passed through optic nerves to the eye. This flux, they believe,

meets with external light to put us into visual contact with external objects. The visual information sent back to the eye through the cone of flux provides representations of species, of those objects, and those representations, in turn, are remanded to the seat of reason in the brain, where they are cognitively judged and stored in memory (Smith 2015, 234).

What a creative perspective on vision! Today, luminous flux refers to the power of a light. There were opposing ideas as well as one controversy related to extromission versus intromission. Extromission involves the eye sending something out to detect an object or a rainbow, and it was the primary belief in medieval times. With intromission, however, something comes from the object and enters the eye. This controversy has been settled, and intromission is the correct mechanism; light rays leave an object and enter the viewer's eye to enable vision. Another development in the Renaissance period was improved glassmaking methods, allowing for more effective eyeglasses for people whose vision was less than perfect. Kepler explained that concave lenses for myopia or nearsightedness were able to correct vision by refraction instead of magnification (Smith 2015, 363).

Retinal Anatomy
I cannot emphasize this enough: the retina is an extension of the brain. The retina is a thin layer at the back of the eye that has a blood supply, called the choroid. The neural retina is a flimsy tissue composed of layers of neurons. In general, neurons are cells in the nervous system that conduct impulses to other neurons in a circuit. They use electrical and chemical signals, known as neurotransmitters, such as glutamate, glycine and dopamine, to communicate with each other.

The three main layers of neurons in the retina are photoreceptors, bipolar cells and retinal ganglion cells, and part of the retinal ganglion cell layer makes up the optic nerve. In order to have vision, a message travels from photoreceptor to bipolar cell to retinal ganglion cell and then through the optic nerve. **Figure 6** displays the basic cell layers of the human retina. The optic nerve then takes retinal signals to the brain for processing.

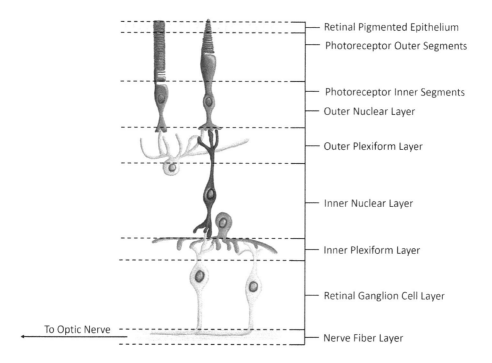

Figure 6: Layers of the retina. Drawing by Bryce Olson

Photoreceptors

Rods and cones are the two classical photoreceptor types that catch light and convert the energy to an electrical signal. Rods are more numerous and spread across the back of the eye, especially the peripheral retina. Cones are more concentrated in the center of the retina at the macula, especially in the center of the macula called the fovea. The **macula** is a yellowish-pigmented area, about two millimeters (mm) in diameter, or one-tenth of the retina. The photosensitive pigments in the human macula belong to a light-absorbing class of molecules called carotenoids. Most carotenoids are found in plants, but the human macula consists of lutein and zeaxanthin (L and Z), which absorb blue light and thus prevent damage to the rest of the retina.

The **fovea** is about 0.4 millimeters in diameter; when attention is fixed on an object, light rays are focused on the fovea. This provides high-acuity vision. There are at least 110 million rods in each human retina, while cones constitute the remaining six million photoreceptors.

The structure of photoreceptor cells is quite unique. Representations of the rod and cone are shown in **Figure 7**. The upper region of the rod cell is called the outer segment, containing about 100 disks or flattened membranous sacs that resemble a stack of coins. The most abundant protein within the disks is rhodopsin, about one million molecules per disk. This protein is essential in capturing light.

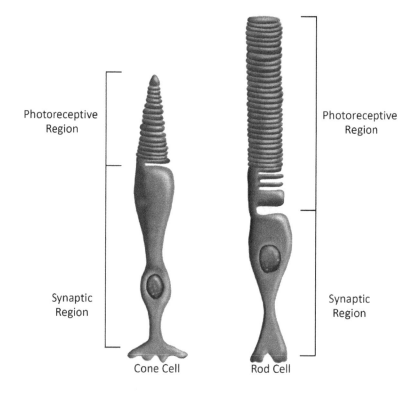

Photoreceptive
Region

Photoreceptive
Region

Synaptic
Region

Synaptic
Region

Cone Cell   Rod Cell

Figure 7: Rod and cone structural details. Drawing by Bryce Olson

Cones were named for their distinctive triangular shape, like an ice cream cone, and they also have membranous disks. In humans, there are three types of cones; they are designated red, green and blue because of the optimum range of wavelengths they absorb. For instance, blue cones absorb wavelengths from 390 to 510 nanometers (nm), with blue being the optimum. Functionally, rods dominate in dim light, while cones operate in brighter light settings and are responsible for color discrimination.

Retinal Pigment Epithelium
Behind the retina lies a single layer of cells, about one million in total, called the retinal pigment(ed) epithelium or RPE. These cells protect the neural retina from potentially damaging light by absorbing stray light rays with their melanin pigment. Another function of RPE cells is to store and re-form vitamin A, which is needed for light detection. The RPE layer also performs a process called phagocytosis, in which cells engulf and degrade old or damaged pieces of photoreceptor cell membranes, known as shed outer segment disks. If these membranes are not digested fully, then they can collect or accumulate gradually, resulting in disease like Stargardt disease.

.

Chapter Four

Eye Doctors, Eye Exams and Patient Advocacy

Eye Doctors

I have met many eye doctors since my diagnosis, mainly because I have moved four times for my career. My eyes have been examined by at least 14 eye doctors: one general ophthalmologist, two optometrists, four low vision specialists and seven retina specialists. Two of these doctors have been guest lecturers in one of my courses, a junior seminar titled Physiology of Vision. I also have recommended three undergraduate students to attend optometry school. I think this qualifies me as an expert on eye doctors.

The title of "eye doctor" refers to either an optometrist or ophthalmologist, and both doctors do eye exams. An optician is not a doctor but a person who fits individuals for glasses, contact lenses and protective eyewear. An **optometrist** has a Doctor of Optometry (O.D.) degree, which requires four or five years of training beyond a Bachelor of Science degree. An optometrist writes prescriptions for eyeglasses or contact lenses and is trained to recognize and treat many eye diseases. It is also possible to get specialized training as an optometrist in the fields of low vision, sports vision, pediatrics or geriatrics. There are 23 optometry schools in the United States, and candidates are selected based on undergraduate grade point average, Optometry Admission Test (OAT) score, and interview (https://www.sco.edu/optometry-schools-in-usa). Getting accepted into optometry school is competitive and comparable to getting into medical school.

An **ophthalmologist** is a medical doctor who has completed a bachelor's degree and four years of medical or osteopathic school, earning a M.D. or D.O. degree. This career path requires a one-year internship in Internal Medicine and three or four years of residency in Ophthalmology. After the residency program, the doctor can select a sub-specialty such as cataracts and refractive surgery, cornea, neuro-ophthalmology, pediatrics or vitreo-retinal surgery. The title of "eye surgeon" applies to most ophthalmologists.

A **retina specialist** is an ophthalmologist who has completed an additional two-year fellowship. Most of the retina specialists I have met are great and knowledgeable doctors. My biggest complaint is the little time that retina specialists spend with their patients—sometimes as little as ten minutes per visit. In only one case did I have an unsatisfactory experience with a retina specialist: he wanted me to perform an unnecessary and expensive test (described in the section on patient advocacy later in this chapter). One bad experience out of 14 doctors is an excellent track record in the medical profession, and it indicates a field of super-competent professionals.

I have heard two common complaints from patients about their eye doctors. Some doctors give the impression, as Dr. Ming Wang (2016) has described of other doctors, that they view their patients as "eyeballs upon which to operate." They consider the patient's condition as an opportunity for surgery rather than a way to improve the patient's well-being. If anyone feels this way about his or her doctor, I advise finding a new one. Even in ophthalmology, bedside manner, or customer service, is important.

The second complaint I have heard is when the patient blames the doctor for his or her change in vision. Let me defend the eye doctors on this point. Doctors have spent years studying how to help patients see better. They know a lot, but the fields of optometry and ophthalmology have limitations. There are many vision disorders that are currently uncorrectable. This is frustrating to the doctor as well as to the patient. Experiencing a vision change is scary, and fear of the unknown creeps into our thoughts.

It is not the doctor's fault when a patient experiences vision changes. Only in rare cases is it the physician's fault, after a procedure goes awry. It is easy to blame the doctor for vision changes, but the real cause is our own eyes. Eyes change over a lifetime. As we age, we may experience the following: decreased focusing ability of the lens, reduced pupil size, increased sensitivity to bright sun and glare, loss of peripheral vision, decreased tear and meibum secretion, and decreased color vision (Haigh 2018). We seem to accept aging changes such as wrinkled skin and age spots, decreased height and increased blood pressure. We need to accept changes in our eyes as normal signs of aging as well.

I have noticed a bit of attitude between optometrists and ophthalmologists, which I mainly attribute to basic competition for patients and their routine care. If ophthalmologists have a thriving practice, they may not need the patient to visit regularly, and the optometrist can monitor the patient. If, however, the ophthalmologists are seeking more income, one common practice is to schedule the patient for two visits per year, performing tests that might be unnecessary. However, Medicare and

Medicaid generally pay for one annual visit. Another difference is that ophthalmologists have a longer period of training, albeit on the whole body rather than on the eye, and sometimes that may affect how they treat optometrists. This is similar to how medical doctors may treat a nurse who has four years of training versus a doctor with 11 or more years of training.

Finally, it is my impression that ophthalmologists are less familiar with low vision doctors, who are optometrists, and the local vision resources for their patients. In my dreams, I wish that when a retina specialist diagnoses a patient with AMD or Stargardt disease, the doctor would provide the patient with an information packet to indicate such things as what to expect and where the patient can access local visual rehabilitation resources (such as social services for the disabled and support groups). My friend with Usher syndrome, Peggy Mitchell, wishes that retina specialists referred patients to The Foundation Fighting Blindness (FFB) at the time of their diagnosis. FFB has about 35 chapters in the United States and raises funds for research to develop treatments for many retinal diseases.

Eye Exams

Each doctor, whether an optometrist, ophthalmologist or retina specialist, examines the patient's eyes and performs some common tests of eye health. Some tests are performed in the light, known as **photopic** vision. Other tests are done in dim light conditions, which is **scotopic** vision. First, the doctor looks for any external problems. Gonioscopy involves inspecting the drainage area of the eye, ensuring that aqueous humor is draining properly. Next, the doctor assesses intraocular pressure and visual acuity. The doctor usually dilates the pupils and examines the inner parts of the eyes with two devices.

Eye pressure, or **intraocular pressure (IOP)**, is measured with a tonometer. Years ago, this test involved a puff of air that many patients found annoying. Newer devices measure IOP in a non-invasive fashion, without the air puff. The normal range of IOP is between 12 and 22 millimeters of mercury (mmHg). A high IOP value is suggestive of glaucoma, which can be treated if detected early.

To determine a patient's **best corrected vision,** or BCV, the patient reads aloud from a Snellen eye chart (refer to Figure 1 in Chapter One). This chart has lines of letters or numbers of different sizes. Acuity of 20/15 indicates sharp vision, or an individual with more functioning retinal cells in the macular region than a subject with 20/20 acuity. The latter value is generally considered normal vision. An acuity test will help the optometrist determine if a patient has a refractive error such as myopia or hyperopia. The doctor also will decide whether correction with eyeglasses or contact lenses is needed.

With a Snellen eye chart, visual acuity is based on units of 20/x, with x being 20, 30, 40, 70, 100, 200 or 400. Let's compare a patient with 20/20 vision (normal vision) to a patient with 20/50 acuity. A person with 20/20 acuity can see this line from 20 feet away, and if they are standing 50 feet from the chart, they can see the 20/50 line. A person with 20/50 acuity cannot see the 20/20 line, nor the 20/25, 20/30 or 20/40 lines. A patient with 20/50 acuity sees things as if they are 30 feet farther away from the object than what the person with 20/20 can see clearly.

The two eyes are examined separately, with the weaker eye being tested first. On prescriptions, the left eye is denoted OS for oculus sinister, and the right eye is OD for oculus dextrus. Opticians are trained to fit patients with eyeglasses or con-

tact lenses; they will either do on-the-job training or get a one-year training certificate. An of-
ten-asked question is, "Will wearing glasses make
my eyes worse?" The answer is no, our eyes change
on their own.

Having a sudden change in vision, perhaps dou-
ble vision (diplopia), is often the first indication
that a patient has diabetes mellitus, and the eye
doctor will refer the patient to other medical professionals to manage this metabolic disorder. Dou-
ble vision also could indicate multiple sclerosis,
thyroid disease or myasthenia gravis.

The doctor will often dilate or enlarge the patient's pupils by applying eye drops with the goal
of viewing the back of the eye. **Dilation** drugs include atropine sulfate, cyclopentolate hydroxide,
phenylephrine hydrochloride and scopolamine hyd-
robromide. Dilation can last more than three hours.

After giving the eyes time to fully dilate, the doctor will view the inner parts of the eye with an **ophthalmoscope** (invented by Hermann von Helmholtz
in 1851) to look at the retina and optic nerve. The
retina appears reddish, and discoloration indicates
disease. A patient with a retinal tear lacks blood
being supplied to that area of the retina, which
leads to cellular death. A detached retina requires
immediate surgery. If detachment is not repaired
quickly, vision loss may be permanent. Damage to
the optic nerve usually indicates glaucoma. The
doctor also will view the blood vessels that supply
bipolar and retinal ganglion cells. Changes in blood
vessels may indicate high blood pressure, diabetes
or age-related macular degeneration (AMD).

Other Vision Tests

There are many other vision tests that may be
performed on a semi-regular basis, but not every
visit. For macular degeneration, the common tests
are intravenous fluorescein angiography, perime-

try (visual field) and optical coherence tomography. **Perimetry** can identify a **scotoma**, an abnormal blind spot in the visual field.

Fluorescien angiography (FA) was mentioned in Chapter One as the definitive test for Stargardt disease. This statement was true in the year 2000, but over the next decade, FA became less popular. What makes it definitive is the silent choroid characteristic. It also detects blood vessels in the retina that leak fluid.

Optical coherence tomography, or OCT, gives a non-invasive cross-sectional image of the retina in extraordinary color. The image shows retinal thinning, or areas where the photoreceptors of the macula used to be, before they died and were removed. The retinal pigment epithelial cell layer is usually disrupted too. Sadly, it is not much to see when the image is black and white. OCT has become a popular test for examining the macula and in some ways is replacing FA. It is less invasive and easier for the patient to tolerate.

The details of a low vision exam are discussed in Chapter Six.

Patient Advocacy

One of my friends suggested that I include a section with all of my advice to patients, rather than spread the pearls of wisdom throughout many chapters of the book. What a great idea!

If I could go back in time and change my interactions with eye doctors, I would do one main thing differently. I would **bring a partner, friend or family member to the doctor appointments to be my advocate**. Perhaps half of my appointments are routine, during which having another person present is not necessary. However, even with my experience as a vision researcher, I cannot accurately predict when a visit will be routine versus non-routine.

When a patient is told devastating news such as "You have macular degeneration," it helps to have a supportive person nearby. As I described in Chapter One, I was alone in a laboratory when my doctor told me my diagnosis over the phone. I was a very independent woman, but I was not prepared for that piece of news. On subsequent doctor visits, as I was processing what they told me, I wish there had been someone else in the room, someone who could have been a witness to the conversation. This would have helped my recollection later ("What did the doctor say when I asked about … ?"). Another person also could have asked questions that had not occurred to me.

When dealing with personal medical information, it is easy to be overwhelmed. My two moments of feeling overwhelmed at eye doctor visits were in March 2000 and June 2011. My first retina specialist visit was when I first used the Amsler grid and discovered a bull's eye blind spot. During what I expected to be a routine optometrist visit in 2011, I was told not to drive home.

For the case of dry AMD or Stargardt disease, I think a change of acuity is a good reason to have an advocate present at an eye doctor visit. With wet AMD, I would recommend having an advocate present at all of the early visits, such as those in which you are deciding which treatment options to pursue.

Examples of Patient Advocacy

I had two visits to Dr. Gass after my diagnosis and asked him several questions. Dr. Gass's answers usually did not satisfy me. First, I asked, "Should I wear sunglasses?" His answer was along the lines of "Sure, it doesn't hurt." This did not seem like a strong endorsement, but I bought a good pair of sunglasses and began wearing them all the time.

Another question I asked was, "Should I limit my exposure to light, as in the experiments with the Stargardt mice?" The Stargardt mouse strain is an animal model of the disease, although the expression of the disease in mouse and human is not identical. This is what is known as a species difference. Dr. Gass replied with the old-school line, "What happens in mice does not necessarily explain what happens in human disease." Initially, I was confused, but after years of working as a scientist, I recognized the truth in his statement. Now, I caution my students not to draw conclusions about human disease from animal studies. Some experiments on animals do replicate what occurs in humans; however, there are many examples of experiments that show moderate or stark differences between the two species.

I asked a question about my symptoms. "Why did my vision halos change color, from yellow to purple?" From his response, it was clear that Dr. Gass believed that I was mistaken, that there was no color change. Years later, I learned why my halo colors changed. I learned a lesson about doctors, too; even world-famous retina specialists do not always fully understand what the patient is experiencing. Over the years, I developed more confidence in myself and continued asking questions.

My most proud example of advocacy relates to the dreaded fluorescein angiogram. I have performed the test twice, in 2000 (for the purpose of diagnosis) and about seven years later. In the first case, I had excellent health insurance, and I do not recall ever seeing the bill. In the second case, my health insurance at the time left a lot to be desired, and I was shocked to get a bill for about $450. I learned my lesson and became a wiser medical service consumer. When my acuity worsened in the year 2011 to 20/110, the retina specialist I visited wanted me to have a third fluorescein angiogram to detect leaking blood vessels. I balked at this request for two reasons. I knew the cost of the test and remembered how much the test bothered me (as if I was being forced to keep my eyes open while bright lights were flashing). More importantly, the FA would not provide much new information. I already knew I had Stargardt disease, and the likelihood that a Stargardt patient has leaking blood vessels is practically nil. I told the doctor that I would not consent to this test and stood my ground.

Chapter Five
Symptoms of Macular Degeneration

Educating oneself about macular degeneration (MD) is a double-edged sword. Although there are many positive aspects of learning, too much knowledge can have a negative impact on a patient's well-being. Learning can be instrumental in helping patients to regain control of their lives. Although I was saddened to learn that there is no effective treatment for Stargardt disease or dry AMD, I was encouraged to hear that patients experience slow degeneration, with symptoms progressing over the course of years.

There is a long list of symptoms associated with macular degeneration. However, the progression of the disease is assessed on an individual basis, with severity and timing of symptoms varying widely between patients. For me, symptoms were not apparent until a number of years after diagnosis. The collection of symptoms is known as a phenotype, or the outward expression of a genetic trait or mutation (after all, one cannot see a genotype).

Before my diagnosis, the acuity in my right eye (OD) was slightly worse than that of my left eye (OS), 20/25 versus 20/20. Fortunately, I was left eye-dominant. Over the next decade, my right eye worsened and then the left eye did. As the disease progressed, my brain adapted to using both eyes equally, or binocular vision.

Central Vision Loss

Macular degeneration results in central vision loss, limiting what can be seen straight ahead within one's visual field. As a reminder, the macula is the center of the retina, and the fovea is the center of the macula. The fovea contains mostly cones for color and fine vision. I first experienced a small amount of central vision loss when my acuity was 20/30. As my condition progressed, so did my loss of central vision. The first time I wrote in my journal about my vision being affected was December 2005, five years after diagnosis. I wrote, "I had trouble reading the *Smithsonian* magazine."

Reading books and music, sewing, driving, playing sports, watching television and attending movies, sports events and theatrical productions, are a handful of activities impacted by loss of central vision. Sewing was never an activity I enjoyed, so that difficulty was not a big deal. It definitely would be dangerous for me to play softball or anything with a fast-moving ball coming near my face.

Central vision loss had the biggest effect on my reading. I was an avid reader in my teenage years and went on to choose a profession that involves a lot of reading. I also am myopic, able to see near objects more clearly than far objects. I currently adjust reading material to point size 14 and need no further optical correction. For some text in a smaller size, I read by bringing the page close to my face. To make reading more comfortable, I require three types of magnifying devices. Due to the fact that I am presbyopic (having the inability to accommodate near objects with age), I also use reading glasses when wearing contact lenses. In essence, the contact lenses provide me with distance vision, while the magnifying reading glasses restore some of my near vision.

On a **computer** or **smart phone**, magnification is rather simple, at least in this technological era. The larger the screen, the more text is displayed.

To read text on paper, like when I grade exams or read a science journal article, I use a hand-held magnifier or a closed circuit television. Both of these devices are described in Chapter Six.

Some social interactions can be affected by central vision loss. Working late one evening at my office desk, my colleague greeted me at the door, about eight feet away. At this point, I knew that the disease was progressing because I could no longer make out any part of his eyes. We were making eye contact, but my eyes were not doing their expected part. Currently, I cannot recognize people's faces or see their facial expressions unless I am less than three feet away.

Monitoring Central Vision Loss
An **Amsler grid** is a simple device that resembles a checkerboard, as shown in Chapter One (Figure 2). It can be magnetically attached to a refrigerator door or transferred to paper. The two forms I have encountered are black grid lines on a white background or white lines on a black background.

Initially, in the center of the grid I saw a blank spot that resembled a ring or bull's eye. In later years, the ring has grown larger, as shown in **Figure 8**. Comparing this image with the one in Chapter One (Figure 3), you can see there is a big difference. This difference illustrates the changes happening to my visual field and indicates progression of the disease.

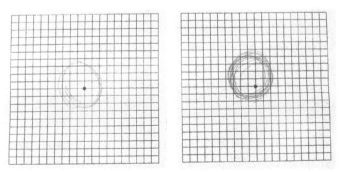

Figure 8: My Amsler grid one year after diagnosis

Instructions to use an Amsler grid, 3-inch x 3-inch version:

1. Test each eye separately by covering the un-used eye. Wear glasses if you normally do.
2. Keep the grid about 14 inches away.
3. Look directly at the dot in the center of the grid.

If a patient notices something new such as blurry lines, dark spots or blank spots on the grid, call a retinal specialist immediately! Amsler grids can be used to identify and monitor the disease, with many doctors encouraging their pa-tients to look at the grid at the same time each day to assess any changes in their vision.

Personally, I do not follow this advice. My dai-ly activities involve reading, and I believe I would notice any visual change. When my vision fell from 20/70 to 20/100, I noticed the changes but was in denial. In my classroom, I believed that my stu-dents were trying to make my life more difficult by selecting small font sizes for their PowerPoint pre-sentations. However, they were following my sug-gestion of using font size no smaller than 24 point for text on a slide. It turned out that my eyes were to blame, not my students.

Distance Vision
As a result of myopia and acuity of 20/110, I can-not see distant objects well. Due to this limitation, navigating new areas is sometimes frustrating, as I may get close to a wall or obstacle before realiz-ing that it is blocking my path.

Halos
I discovered I had a blind spot or **scotoma** using the Amsler grid in 2000 at my first retinal examination. Then I began seeing this image (or lack of sight)

more often. The halo was not the classic blind spot that everyone has, which is due to the optic nerve having no photoreceptors at that location. Instead, what I observed was in the shape of a bull's eye target. In the center of my visual field I saw a ring that shimmered. In my journal entry from September 2001, I wrote that I had "many halos" and connected them to lack of sleep. As the disease progressed, the tiny ring became thicker. When the halo first appeared, it was distracting. I described it as a donut hole that I could see through. Over the years, the hole in the center reduced in size, eventually filling in to become my blind spot.

At first the halo appeared when my eyes were tired, so I started to associate it with eye fatigue. Gradually, the halo became more prominent to me. About ten years after my diagnosis, I could see it nearly every day, even when I had a full night's sleep.

Early on, the color of my blind spot was distinctly yellow. Why yellow? Maybe because I was afraid, and yellow is the color I associate with fear. I had never before "seen" blind spots, and at this point I was seeing them once to several times per day. In the next year, my spots changed to a purple color, and on rare occasions they were green.

Why does the halo have a color? I think it is due to my brain's attempt to fill in the blank spaces in my visual field. Although annoying, I find it less bothersome than having a blank spot without color. Over the years, my halo has blended into the scenery. It is still present; however, my brain has adapted to suppress it.

I want to clarify that my blind spots are not the same as afterimages, which are normal physiological phenomena. Afterimages last about 30 seconds and occur after exposure to bright light, such as a camera flash or vehicle headlights. They are due to the activation and saturation of photoreceptors following exposure to a stimulus. The image remains in our visual field, even after our eyes close. As the photoreceptors begin to "recover," the afterimage will subside, and the photoreceptors reset for the next stimulus. In other words, our eyes and brain continue working even after we shut our eyes. Although I see afterimages, I also experience halo blind spots.

Visual Field

Fortunately, my peripheral or side vision is unaffected by macular degeneration, but some patients do experience losses in their peripheral vision. With my peripheral vision, I am able to detect nearby movement, such as a squirrel darting up a tree or a person walking by. Both of my eyes are equally competent, with my peripheral vision being similar on the left and right sides. In my visual field, I can detect moving objects more easily than stationary ones.

Night Blindness

Night blindness is the subjective sensation of difficulty identifying objects under conditions of low illumination. I discovered this issue about five years after my diagnosis, when my acuity was 20/40. I began to see poorly in low light settings like a dim movie theater, dark restaurant or outside at night. Night driving is probably not safe for me; walking in the dark, though, is not too bad. I rarely trip, so my mobility is unaffected by Stargardt disease. Mobility is generally affected when blind spots begin to encroach upon the peripheral field of vision.

Light Sensitivity

There is variability in this characteristic, with some patients being more sensitive to bright light than others. In my case, I think it was more psychosomatic in the sense that I believed I was light sensitive after reading articles about light damaging the retina. I imagined that every bright light was causing further harm to my photoreceptors. For several years, I put on sunglasses before leaving any building. It reached a ridiculous point where I insisted that no photographs could be taken of me unless I was wearing dark sunglasses. I even got angry when a friend snapped a flash photo of me unprepared (i.e., not wearing protection).

Color Deficiency

I discovered this condition later than the other symptoms, during a low vision exam (20/100 acuity). Dr. Prischak was wearing a tie and asked me how many shades (hues) of green I could see. I answered three, and he told me that his tie had five shades of green. I was stunned, and we politely argued about it until I accepted this truth.

In 2015, while at a vision research conference, I had the opportunity to assess my color discrimination with the Cone Contrast Test (CCT), which was the same test that Air Force pilots take. It gave me a cone-specific numeric score relative to a person with normal color vision. I learned that my sensitivity to red, green and blue hues was 10%, 50% and 75%, respectively, of normal. In other words, I could barely see any red letters, but my ability to detect blue letters was only slightly reduced.

Charles Bonnet Syndrome (CBS)

I have read about this condition in an introductory neuroscience textbook and have spoken with a few people who have experienced it. A patient with CBS sees images or hallucinations that are not there. They seem real, like a dream, but it is not the eyes that are seeing them, and patients are awake when they appear. The brain is no longer receiving any external visual input but instead becomes overactive and produces images. About 10% of visual-ly-impaired individuals, especially older patients, experience them. They differ from psychotic hal-lucinations because the images do not instruct or interact with the patient (Sacks 2009).

Oliver Sacks has described the Charles Bonnet syndrome. Sacks, a renowned neurologist, wrote case studies of his patients and himself. One of these studies involved treating some patients with L-DOPA, a drug typically used to treat Parkinson's disease. This story would later be portrayed in the movie *Awakenings*. Sacks (2009) claimed that only 1% of patients actually report images to their doctors, mainly for fear of being declared mentally unsta-ble or insane or being diagnosed with dementia. Patients might describe their images as watching a silent movie, as the images appear suddenly but do not fade away as in a dream. Frequent themes are deformed faces, cartoons or a television screen. Sacks himself saw geometric shapes like tiles.

Other Symptoms
Some people with macular degeneration can see better on cloudy days than on sunny days. This can occur due to photophobia, or an extreme sensi-tivity to light.

Summary of Symptoms
As with many diseases, not all patients with mac-ular degeneration experience all of the just-men-tioned symptoms. However, other serious eye prob-lems may occur such as cataracts, glaucoma or diabetic retinopathy. Unfortunately, it is possible to have more than one vision problem.

Causes of Symptoms
There are both genetic and environmental causes of macular degeneration. **Genetic causes** are still under investigation. Currently, genes known to be

associated with MD include ATP-binding cassette in the retina (ABCA4, previously ABCR), elongation of very long chain fatty acids 4 (ELOVL4), and complement factor H (CFH). Identifying the gene that contains a mutation is an active area of clinical research. Environmental risk factors of MD include smoking, excessive sun or ultraviolet light exposure, vascular disease and nutritional status. Inflammation in the retina is another factor that is believed to contribute to AMD.

Types of Macular Degeneration
There are at least three types of macular degeneration. Diagnosis is based on what the clinician observes at the macula as well as the age of the patient. In ophthalmic terms, any age before age 50 is considered juvenile. If the patient is over age 50, it is usually called age-related macular degeneration (AMD or ARMD). The greater the age, the higher the likelihood that a person develops AMD. If the patient is under age 50, the term "macular dystrophy" is often used, or "juvenile macular degeneration." Diseases of this category include Stargardt disease, fundus flavimaculatus, Best's vitelliform macular dystrophy, Doyne's honeycomb retinal dystrophy and Sorsby's fundus dystrophy.

AMD affects 50 million people worldwide including 15 million Americans. This condition is more common in people who smoke, consume a high fat diet, and are of Caucasian or North European descent. AMD is categorized into dry and wet types, with the dry (atrophic) type being more common. Further classification signifies its progression with early and advanced stages. Approximately 1.7 million Americans have advanced forms of the disease. One type is known as wet (exudative) AMD, or choroidal neovascularization (CNV). This means that there is new blood vessel formation at the back of the retina. It also may involve detachment of the retinal pigment epithelial (RPE) cells. The advanced dry form is called geographic atrophy (GA).

Dry AMD is more common. This type has no effective treatment; doctors recommend a healthy diet with vitamins and antioxidants. In the case of wet AMD, blood vessels leak fluid and scar, new blood vessels form in a process called angiogenesis, and the retina is damaged. The wet form of AMD is more problematic, as blood vessels become abnormal and leak. If wet AMD is not treated, the prognosis is progressive loss of vision within one year. The average age of diagnosis of wet AMD is 71 years.

Stargardt disease (STGD) affects around 30,000 Americans and is a form of macular degeneration that affects people younger than 50. The main differences between dry AMD and Stargardt disease are age of onset and genetic influence.

Why Does the Macula Degenerate?
This is the $64,000 question, right? The biological answer is that photoreceptor cells die. Cells of the retina usually last for a lifetime, so this death is premature. Cones are primarily located in the macula, but both cones and rods die. Whether it is rods or cones that die first is less important relative to treatment options. When death occurs, cells induce their neighbors to die. In some cases, RPE cells die first, which then leads to photoreceptor cell death. The area of the macula that is damaged is as small as four millimeters, equivalent to the diameter of a spaghetti noodle. That's a tiny yet important area!

Cell death is a vast subject. If an injury occurs such as a knife piercing the skin, cell death is called necrosis, a normal process where damaged cells are removed from the body. The other type of cell death is apoptosis, in which death signals appear to come from inside the cell or neighboring cells.

Why do photoreceptor cells die in macular degeneration? Most likely and in simple terms, it is related to apoptosis and the macula area having high oxygen demands. More oxygen utilization means more oxygen damage, or oxidative stress. Patients develop deposits of yellowish material called **drusen**, which are also found in skin (called age spots), and much research has been done to determine whether drusen have an influence on the disease (cause or effect). Drusen contain waste products, and one of the main "players" is a molecule called **lipofuscin**, which seems correlated to cell death.

How many photoreceptor cells die? Geller and Sieving (1993, 1521) have tested Stargardt patients to answer this question. They demonstrated that about 90% of photoreceptors are lost (85% to 92% in the central fovea) when central vision loss is apparent. This study examined patients with visual acuities widely ranging from 20/30 to 20/100. In another study, Geller, Sieving and Green (1992, 474) found that performance for a visual task was not impacted (decreased) until the retina was 88% degenerated. As for implications, keeping more photoreceptors alive should maintain or preserve central vision.

Treatments
First, there are no approved treatments for dry AMD and Stargardt disease. This is incredibly frustrating for the majority of macular degeneration patients. However, science has told us one important action, although it is not a treatment per se. In 2001, a landmark study called Age-Related Eye Disease Study (AREDS no. 8) was published about AMD. Study participants had early signs of AMD and took a combination of antioxidants (vitamin C, vitamin E and beta carotene) and zinc for at least six years. This study found that the oral supple-

ment delayed progression from early to advanced AMD (AREDS Research Group, 2001). Since then, substances such as lutein and zeaxanthin (known as macular pigments) and saffron have been added to the formula, with the intention of delaying AMD progression. Quite a large number of eye supplements based on AREDS are on the market and available at any pharmacy, and every eye doctor I have met recommend them to their patients with AMD.

I took some version of the macular pigment formula soon after I was diagnosed, then stopped for years. By 2014, I resumed taking this formula, and I added saffron and astaxanthin around 2018. Although it is my opinion as a patient who is a vision researcher (anecdotal evidence), I think taking this formula has helped my vision. I wish I had not stopped taking them for those years, which was at a time when my vision loss did progress.

For those with wet AMD, effective treatments have been available since 2007. The current treatment involves the injection of an antibody that inhibits a molecule called vascular endothelial growth factor, or VEGF. These injections into the eye are scheduled with a retina specialist every four to six weeks, with promising results. There are three effective anti-VEGF drugs (Avastin, Lucentis and Eylea). There is much discussion about which drug to use and the frequency of injections, and I will stay away from clinical recommendations. These drugs have demonstrated improved vision for many clinical trial participants. After following a monthly treatment regimen, patients gained the ability to discriminate, on average, eight letters of an ETDRS chart better than baseline acuity (Angiogenesis Foundation 2017, 12).

Chapter Six
Low Vision and Assistive Devices

What Is Low Vision?

In the first article I read about AMD in 2000, Kals and Lauerman (2000, 81) suggested asking an ophthalmologist about a "low vision" specialist. I had no idea what low vision was then. I learned about it years later.

Low vision is a general term referring to reduced vision that is not correctable with glasses, surgery or treatment (Judith A. Read Low Vision Services brochure 2018). This can relate to visual acuity or visual field and results in impaired function. One number associated with low vision is acuity of 20/70. Low vision is not a single disease and can include a variety of visual disorders, such as central vision loss (macular degeneration), peripheral vision loss (retinitis pigmentosa), diabetic retinopathy, cataract and glaucoma. According to Wikipedia, over 3.4 million Americans have low vision, which is having distance visual acuity of 20/70 or worse in the best-corrected eye.

Unfortunately, due to a lack of patient education being offered by medical professionals, many people have never heard of low vision and wouldn't know they could benefit from consulting a low vision doctor. At what point does a patient need a low vision consultation? A good rule of thumb is when the patient is experiencing vision changes that are affecting daily tasks.

When my visual acuity reached 20/40, I was experiencing trouble doing some daily tasks. Before then, I did not need low vision aids, but it became increasingly useful as my acuity worsened. Low vision became a new branch of knowledge to explore.

I discovered low vision about six years after my diagnosis. I was living in Jackson, Tennessee, and trying to make a place for myself in the community. In a truly fortuitous moment, I was watching a Lambuth University basketball game while sitting next to a colleague from the Department of Education. I felt comfortable sharing my vision story with her and relating how my reading duties were taking much longer than they used to. She told me about a child with vision problems who had been sent to a local organization called the STAR Center.

Although I doubted that this center would be appropriate for adults, I was wrong. The STAR Center, or Special Technology Access Resource, was founded in 1988 by Margaret and Chuck Doumitt. Two of their children had been diagnosed with Batten disease, a condition that leads to blindness, seizures and loss of motor skills. Margaret decided to bring the assistive technology to her children instead of moving to where such technology already existed. The center grew dramatically in West Tennessee, offering many services such as art and music therapies, vocational training and vision services, which include low vision and orientation and mobility (O & M) training. O & M training provides skills in traveling independently, such as with a cane, for patients having visual field (peripheral) deficits. Through grants, fundraising and advertising, the center drew more clients, numbering 17,000 in 2004, serving any type of disability. It became the largest assistive technology center in the United States.

I scheduled a low vision consultation in 2008. At that time, my OD (right eye) acuity was 20/160 and OS (left eye, dominant) acuity was 20/40. I was complaining about having difficulty reading text-books and newspapers, which led to eye strain. The optometrist recommended two items, a hand-held magnifier and closed-circuit television (CCTV), which I still use regularly.

A Low Vision Exam

A low vision examination is specific to a patient's eye condition, remaining vision and goals for im-proving daily activities. Maybe the patient is hav-ing trouble reading, sewing, driving or playing sports. The doctor tests the ability to see details and evaluates visual fields as well as general eye health. Some tests are done monocularly (one eye at a time) and others binocularly (both eyes to-gether). The purpose of the exam is to identify aids to assist patients in their daily living. These aids include prescribed special optical devices and non-optical solutions. Most patients are referred to a low vision doctor by another eye doctor.

I think Freeman and Jose (1991, 6) set the stage for appropriate expectations: "First, you must real-ize there are no miracles. Your lost vision cannot be restored. Low vision is a rehabilitation process. That means you are going to be taught how to effec-tively use your remaining vision." This exam is not for obtaining a new prescription for eyeglasses.

The goal of a low vision exam is to provide the patient with solutions to daily problems for a bet-ter quality of life. A low vision doctor is an optom-etrist with special training. During an exam, the doctor performs a visual acuity test, exposing one line at a time and encouraging guessing. It is okay for the patient to move their eyes around, perhaps viewing around a blind spot. This involves a chart with more lines than the standard Snellen chart, including lines for 20/80, 20/110, 20/120 and 20/150. The most common kind used for this purpose is an ETDRS (Early Treatment Diabetic Retinopathy Study) chart. There are five letters on each row.

The doctor assesses visual field, scotoma (blind spot) and distortion. Kinetic perimetry is a type of visual field test in which the patient fixes his or her eyes on center, a white dot appears from any direction, and the individual is asked to identify when the dot comes into his or her field of vision.

The low vision doctor assesses contrast sensitivity (CS), which gives a more complete measure of spatial vision than acuity. Just as hearing tests use varying sound frequencies and intensities, so "contrast sensitivity tests use contrast and single spatial frequencies to measure visual sensitivity to complex targets" (Ginsberg 1983, 17). A low threshold translates to high sensitivity. Studying how quickly Air Force pilots identified targets, clinicians concluded that 20/20 acuity was not enough and that contrast sensitivity was more predictive of visual performance. The same tool used to select pilots was then applied to candidates for driver's licenses.

A low vision doctor typically introduces the patient to such devices as magnifiers, prisms, high-powered reading glasses, telescopes and electronic magnification systems. The doctor may instruct the patient to experiment with eccentric viewing, or to practice focusing on objects with a peripheral part of the eye rather than the central portion or fovea. Another example is when a schoolteacher is writing on the chalkboard but, out of the corner of his or her eye, is simultaneously looking at two students passing notes in class (Freeman and Jose 1991, 45).

A Change in Mindset

As explained in Chapter Five, many symptoms occur with macular degeneration. The next step is finding solutions to improve the remaining vision. I used to be able to do certain tasks easily with my vision, but later I could not. I was presented with a problem: did I want to continue not being able to do these tasks, clinging to the memory of what I used to be able to do, or did I want to find new ways to accomplish them? I chose function over non-function. I found assistive devices that allowed me to do many of the things I wanted to do.

Technology is meant to make things easier and faster. It is for everyone, not only the disabled community. Assistive technology, on the other hand, is any device or aid that provides access toward independence. I wouldn't consider myself a Luddite, someone who is opposed to technological change, but I am slow to accept it in my own life. It took me years to adapt to using the hand-held magnifier and CCTV. It is ironic that these two devices are the ones I currently use the most in my daily activities.

Local blind groups offer various opportunities for clients to learn about technology to assist visually-impaired people. The Keystone Blind Association (KBA) offers a Tech-Talk meeting each month. Bob George of KBA wrote, in a personal communication to me,

At this interaction, a qualified leader directs a discussion about cutting-edge technology available to help those with visual impairments. Examples of this technology are often made available for clients to interact with and experience first-hand to personally evaluate their low-vision value.

If there are no local blind assistive organizations, consider visiting the website of the Council of Citizens with Low Vision International (CCLVI, www.cclvi.org), which has a mission of education and advocacy.

Tips for Improved Daily Living
There are some simple steps to improve vision.

First, good **lighting** is crucial. Providing more light intensity often helps to discriminate things in the visual scene around you. I would suggest looking into direct or task lighting and experimenting with different light intensities. Lighting is very individual; what is good for one person is not necessarily good for another (Freeman and Jose 1991, 63). Since **fluorescent lights** bother my eyes, I try to avoid them. Sometimes I can detect a flicker that reminds me of an annoying strobe light.

Solutions for Daily Tasks

Some of the items mentioned here can be found in low vision catalogs. Anyone can use these aids in daily living; one does not have to be blind or experience low vision to benefit from using a device. The two most popular low vision catalogs are from MaxiAids and LS&S (Learning Sight & Sound).

There are many **inexpensive aids** to allow for better function, such as lined paper, colored labels and large alphabet letters that can be used as labels. If a patient is having trouble writing checks, especially with finding the signature line, one simple tool is a signature guide.

Useful Tools for Low Vision

Protective lenses are helpful. Sunglasses increase contrast and reduce glare, thus improving clarity. My advice about **sunglasses** is simple: wear them! Invest in a pair of sunglasses or get eyeglasses that darken in bright light. I wear sunglasses nearly every day and rarely go outside on a sunny day without them. Polarized lenses reduce glare.

I personally recommend spending a little more money on a pair that is higher quality, with advanced blue-blocking features. Blue wavelengths are most damaging to the retina, and people with light-colored irises, which absorb fewer light rays, experience more light penetrating their retinas. I would rather spend $120 than $15 to block the most damaging rays. However, if you tend to lose your sunglasses on a regular basis, then cheaper ones might be the best option.

When I moved to Manhattan, I wore my sunglasses devoutly. I would put them on in the elevator, before I entered the lobby. The doorman commented on a rainy day, about three months after I moved in, that it was the first time he had seen me without my sunglasses, and he didn't know that I had blue eyes.

Glasses with colored filters are interesting tools. These non-prescription glasses have colored lenses to absorb short wavelengths, which reduces glare. The more common colors are yellow, light amber and orange. The yellow filter blocks blue wavelengths, which is useful for outdoor activities, including hunting. One of the big manufacturers is NOIR. I use my yellow pair on gray, rainy or snowy days.

Large print material is a growing category, including books, playing cards, telephone dials and calculators. Large print books typically use size 16-point font, and common publishers are Thorndike Press and The Large Print Book Company (specializing in the classics). Patients with 20/100 or better acuity can read these. My only complaint about large print books is that the figure legends are rarely enlarged. Why would you enlarge the text of the entire book but leave that part out?

Books in other formats are useful. **Audiobooks** are available in various ways. The National Library Service for the Blind and Print Disabled (NLS) offers access to books, magazines and music scores (www://nlsbard.loc.gov). The Braille and Audio Reading Download (BARD) program has over 115,000 audio and Braille fiction and nonfiction available. There is even a mobile app for iOS and Android. It is free once you have a membership. One private company that sells audiobooks is Audible.

Kindle and Kindle Paperwhite (by Amazon) are electronic reading devices, costing around $130, with a front light design that reduces shine and makes reading easier. Purchased books can be downloaded from a website and then viewed on the Kindle device screen. The difference between the two types is number of pixels.

Smart devices, including phones and tablets, are good to use. One of my friends drove me to a phone store and helped me select an Apple 4S iPhone in 2011. Its enlarged text settings made reading texts enjoyable rather than something I dreaded. There are so many features on this phone! Probably my favorite feature is Notepad, but I like asking Siri various questions aloud and hearing an audio response. A smart tablet such as an iPad is very useful, as the size of the content on the screen can be easily manipulated with two fingers. I actually use my iPad more than my computer for website searches.

In terms of **computer accessibility**, there have been huge strides made with computers and other smart devices in the past two decades. Apple/Macintosh lead the industry in this area, although some people claim (in 2018) that Microsoft has better accessibility. I'll let the reader decide.

When using a personal computer, one simple thing that can be changed is the color contrast of the display. As mentioned in Chapter One, when I was in graduate school, my sister suggested changing the text color of my document files. I tried this strategy with my dissertation chapters. My favorite colors then were green text on a black background and yellow text on a blue background. In addition, I have used various large monitors for my work. A larger screen offers more text (or figure) to view without having to move the cursor. Unlike television, where the entire picture shrinks on a smaller screen, with computers you can see a portion of the whole picture.

Google Doc was a software program that presented me with many error messages when I attempted to open it with Microsoft. Finally, I switched to a Macintosh computer and never got this message again. Hopefully Windows has improved its software by now, so that this problem has been corrected. The level of accessibility in computers changes regularly: one year Company A is best; another year it's Company B. I suppose that is what drives innovation.

Assistive Devices for Low Vision
In general, assistive devices allow low vision patients to perform activities that would otherwise be difficult, or even impossible, without them. Although I can put some reading materials close to my face to read, this step is awkward and not comfortable. There are many assistive devices for low vision, creating a bewildering number of choices in a catalog. This is why it is helpful to ask your low vision doctor for recommendations of appropriate items for the individual patient. One item may be perfect for me, but another item may be better for my low vision friend.

The **aspheric hand-held magnifier** is my favorite device; it is made by Eschenbach Optik of America, Inc. and costs about $125 (www.eschenbach.com), as shown in **Figure 9**. I use it nearly every day. When I am in public, I use it at restaurants to read the menu. I use it to read the computer screen if I cannot enlarge the text. Its dimensions are 4 inches x 3 inches (100 mm x 75 mm), with 2.8x magnification. Since it weighs 177 grams (my sunglasses weigh 37 grams), I do not carry it around my neck.

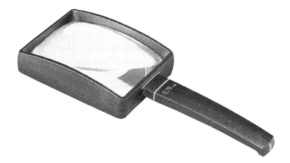

Figure 9: Aspheric hand-held magnifier, Eschenbach model 2655-175

I found a cute way to carry it for all of its use outside my home: I put it in an oven mitt. When I dropped my first magnifier, the glass lens did not break but the damaged handle was not functional. When my second magnifier fell off of the couch and broke, there was no saving it. I immediately ordered a replacement magnifier through my employer. Having two magnifiers is convenient, as I can leave one at work and one at home, risking less breakage upon transport.

Before a low vision doctor recommended the Eschenbach device, I had purchased a smaller magnifying glass. It worked for some of my reading tasks, but it was not the strength or size that I needed. I noted in my journal in 2006 that I still could not read a textbook in the classroom with it, and my solution was to raise the book closer to my face.

There are also many small hand-held devices, some of which have a light. I keep a lighted device in my purse for dark-lit situations like restaurants. However, the visual field is so small (one inch) that it takes a long time to read an entire menu. Sometimes I resort to asking the waiter for the specials instead of attempting to carefully read the list myself.

CCTV, closed-circuit television system, is not a television but a camera attached to a monitor. It works by placing the object or reading material beneath the camera, then selecting settings such as color (black and white, color, yellow, green). The device auto-focuses, and the contents are displayed on the monitor at varying sizes of up to a maximum of 20x. The last step is to zoom in or zoom out. Some products have a tray that moves the material; moving the tray is easier than physically moving a book placed above the tray. Placing a piece of plexiglass above a large book will help to give a flatter surface for more legibility.

The two products I have used are Topaz (Freedom Scientific) and Acrobat (22-inch LCD with X-Y table, Enhanced Vision), the latter as shown in **Figure 10**. The cost of a 19-inch color product is about $3,000, and this was the item I requested for work accommodations. I use it to read books, journal articles and papers in regular-size print. At home, I use it to read bank statements, bills, newsletters, recipes and personal notes. Some of my relatives and friends have figured out that their handwriting is too small or illegible for a low vision person to read, and thus they write larger than normal or type their message. However, not everyone has taken notice of my needs.

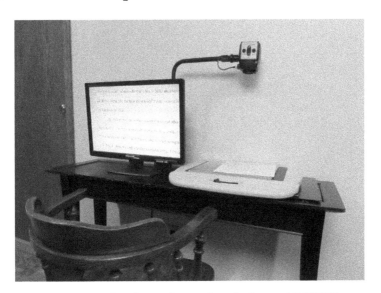

Figure 10: Closed-circuit television (CCTV)

In my experience, a nearby lamp plus the overhead ceiling light should be on when using the CCTV. Having only a single light source may not be sufficient for viewing.

Bioptic telescopic glasses have helped me. Refer to Chapter Twelve for a full description of a spectacle telescope known as bioptic glasses.

Other devices vary. In 2019, NuEYES came on the market, which is a pair of smart glasses that magnify up to 12x and cost around $6,000 (www.nueyes.com). Another recent device is called Orcam My Eye (Explore.orcam.com) that allows the user to read text, recognize faces and money and identify objects, products and colors. It costs about $3,000.

Chapter Seven

Daily Living

As Mogk and Mogk (2003, 14) point out, "Eyesight affects every aspect of life: mobility, physical activity, communication, appearance, perception, self-esteem, and psychological health." When vision loss progresses slowly, the patient has time to adjust to changes. I remember what I used to be able to see, although as more time passes, I am less aware of it all. This chapter details some of the adjustments that I made as my vision deteriorated. They are organized into categories of personal care, activities in the home, activities outside the home and miscellaneous. The tasks are highlighted with boldface to emphasize the number of things that low vision impacts.

One of the adjustments in daily living relates to **learning**. I had always been a very strong visual learner, but without good vision, I had to use other means. Now I use auditory learning and kinesthesia (awareness of the body's position and movement in space). I've come to rely on other senses much more than my sight. In essence, it is switching to alternative ways of collecting information. Freeman and Jose (1991, 37) note that patients "also learn how to use the information they receive through their other senses to supplement the reduced amount of information they obtain visually."

This adjustment for me was a matter of, "Gee, this task used to be a lot easier when I could see better." John Hull (1990, 78) describes "sighted people as rushing around and trying to do more things, while blind people set aside time to do tasks. They cannot increase the pace," but they can be happy about reaching goals.

I wonder why our world insists on using such small print? I would like to believe that only a few tasks are impaired by my vision, but that would be a lie. So many tasks require fine acuity. An Eschenbach brochure "Better Vision, Better Life" (2010, 4) describes it perfectly:

> Why can't newspaper print be larger? Perhaps you know the problem all too well. In your everyday life, you are constantly faced with situations where important information, such as price tags or labels, are presented in a form which is too small to read. You experience similar difficulties when trying to read bus or train timetables. Much of the information we encounter at home or when we're out and about is difficult or even impossible to read because the size of the point is simply too small.

Personal Care. I began **applying makeup** only a few years before my vision diagnosis. I can't read the names of the colors of lipsticks because of the tiny print size. I can, however, distinguish if they are in the pink, red or warm category, so I devised a system. I keep three lipsticks together: one neutral, one warm and one pink/red shade. From these I choose one that complements my outfit that morning. Nonetheless, makeup mistakes are common, occurring about two times per month (especially with mascara and confusing lip liner for eye liner). I should probably look more carefully in the mirror when I finish applying it, as there may be lipstick on my teeth or cheek color that needs more blending. Sometimes, my co-workers and even students have pointed out my mistakes, but I have learned that most are not worth worrying about.

Another thing that became more challenging was painting my toenails. As my disease progressed, seeing my toes was difficult. I realized it's easier to just pay for a **pedicure**.

Activities inside the Home. Fortunately, in the kitchen, my **cooking** practices did not have to change much. I tend to lean over the stove to look closely at the dials, memorize common settings (medium heat), and use additional lighting. To read a recipe that I have not yet memorized, I use a closed circuit television (CCTV). To read directions or ingredients on a can or package of food I use a hand-held magnifier. **Misidentifying food items** occurs when I share a kitchen. I have accidentally put lentils in my yogurt, mistaking them for granola when the bags were sitting next to each other on the counter. So again, organization is key (now we keep the lentils on a shelf instead of a counter).

One thing that seemed ridiculous to me was that I addressed and stamped **envelopes** upside down. I could not tell which side was up! After making that mistake more than once, I learned to check before writing on the envelope. **Paying bills** is much faster when I use a CCTV or pay them online using magnification commands on a computer. Clipping **coupons** became a chore because the only way I could read the expiration dates was to use a CCTV. At some point, I wondered whether the monetary savings was worth the effort. When **watching television**, I moved my seat closer.

Reading for enjoyment is one of my regular activities. When my acuity was 20/40, I struggled to read newspapers. As my vision worsened, reading wasn't fun anymore and became a dreaded chore. Hull (1990, 52) describes it this way: "To read the whole of this book, at this speed, will take an age. Very well. I will not even attempt it." There was a time in my life when I stopped reading for enjoyment, and the only time I read was for work. Henry Grunwald (1999, 91) could not read book titles at the bookstore. I shared his sentiment: "Books haunt me."

Although reading takes more time than it used to, I still prefer the tactile experience of reading a book with my eyes and hands. Once I discovered large print books, I resumed reading for enjoyment. Finding large print books is not so simple. Most commercial bookstores are a big disappointment. Either they have no large print books at all, or their few large print books are mixed in with the regular sections. I had success with some stores that sell used large print books. One store has a large print section with five shelves of fiction and one shelf (40 books) of nonfiction. There are some public libraries with a wide selection of large print books: the public library in Meadville, Pennsylvania, had three rows of large print fiction and almost one full row of large print nonfiction. However, my neighborhood library is geared toward children's books and only has about a dozen large print books for adult readers. Overall, finding large print books is a hit-or-miss endeavor.

With acuity of 20/110, the size of large print books is close to the threshold of my reading ability. If my vision worsens, I will switch from large print books to audiobooks. I am using my Audible account more often, but some steps are hard to perform because of the small print of the application, which, like ride applications, are not enlargeable. There are many book titles that I cannot find in large print or audio format, and thus I read regular print books with a CCTV.

I used to enjoy putting **jigsaw puzzles** together, which gave me time to work my brain and reflect on my life. As my vision worsened, some puzzles became incredibly difficult to complete. Eventually

I donated them to others rather than spend additional hours to complete them. I kept a few of my favorite puzzles.

One of the places I lived had different keys for the front and side doors. Neither door had good street lighting, so I often struggled to **find the right key** to open the door. My solution was to add colored and different shaped labels (for example, a blue semicircle for front door) to my keys. This seemed easier than carrying a flashlight with me or leaving a house light on when I left for work each morning.

Activities outside the Home. On sunny days, I wear sunglasses and a brimmed hat to protect my eyes from glare. On overcast days, I select a pair of yellow-tinted glasses (I'm sure my neighbors think I am much more fashionable than I really am).

Scanning a room to find a certain person can be hard. This is a useful skill in a restaurant or auditorium. It is also useful for networking in a work or career advancement environment (when people scan the room to identify their next conversation partner). The solution to this problem is either finding a different networking method or asking someone to look around for me (for instance, "Do you see Susan?"). **Reading the time** on a clock or watch is sometimes difficult, depending on the hands and numbers contrasting with the background. Most digital clocks have tiny displays.

On numerous occasions, I have deposited checks into my bank account with mistakes in the subtotal. Although I tell the clerk that it is a math error, it is usually because I read the numbers incorrectly due to my vision. Feigning errors is easier than explaining my vision limitations to the clerk.

Another early adjustment I made outside the home was **reading menus** at a restaurant, which sometimes have small print. I regularly carry hand-held and lighted magnifiers in my purse. On rare occasions, a server has commented on it, but it doesn't feel socially awkward. When a magnifying device is not handy, I have asked the server about the specials or his or her favorite item. I've found that interacting with the serving staff is usually successful and that I do not necessarily need to mention my vision status. Occasionally, I look for a menu online before I visit a new restaurant. I wish more restaurants had large print menus; Cracker Barrel is one of the chains that does and all a customer needs to do is ask for it.

Reading concert programs or **church bulletins** is difficult. Once I find a church service that meets my needs, I ask a greeter if he could request that the church secretary make some large print bulletins. Some congregations with many elderly members already do this, so I may not be the first person to need this accommodation.

Shopping. When I am at a **checkout area** of a retail store and paying with a debit or credit card, it is difficult to read the small print instructions. A friend suggested an easy remedy when I cannot read the fine print of a receipt at a store. I say, "I forgot my reading glasses in the car." This is a socially acceptable reason for me to struggle when reading a receipt. Now that I am old enough to have presbyopia, no one challenges my statement.

Grocery stores appeal to the vision of shoppers. Visiting one store regularly makes it easier since I can learn where items are located, and some grocery chains have similar layouts and items. Still, I commonly make mistakes in making selections. I might grab the wrong type of orange juice (high pulp versus no pulp) or an avocado from the organic section instead of the regular produce. Usually, it's only a minor annoyance. However, buying the wrong item needed for a recipe is a bigger issue and then I have to go back to the store to get what I need. I tend to buy the same items on a regular basis so I don't have to read a lot of labels and prices. As with makeup and coupons, it's just not worth spending a lot of time on these tasks.

Shopping for clothes can be hard with low vision because stores rotate their items. It seems like every time I shop, the arrangement is new. New areas require more scanning. The main issue I have with clothes is reading sizes on labels. Now I bring a hand-held magnifier or a friend.

Transportation and Mobility. My walking ability has not been affected by my vision; I do not need any walking devices. For people with peripheral vision loss, mobility is the biggest challenge, and mobility training often involves canes or a guide dog.

I received a gift of a visually-impaired **cane with a red tip**, which indicates that the user can see some things. Totally blind persons use a white cane. My cane folds into a size that tucks into a bag or purse. This has been useful when I travel alone through a large airport. It's sometimes hard to read the ticket, so I routinely ask the ticketing clerk for the pertinent information and then memorize it. Once, a clerk told me to look at my boarding pass. Unfortunately, it was not an ideal situation to explain that I have low vision, but obviously I wouldn't have asked if I could have read it myself! I noticed on subsequent trips as soon as the ticketing agents saw the cane, their demeanor improved. Airport staff are just nicer to people who need some assistance. In current years, my frustration at airports is limited to not being able to read the monitors that provide departure and baggage information. In those cases, I ask someone else who is looking for their flight to look for mine.

I think it creates good traveler karma!

In terms of **driving**, it took me many years to accept that it is okay to be a non-driver. Chapters Eight and Nine specifically address this issue.

Miscellaneous. When choosing which **sports** to play, the phrase "do no harm" has become my mantra. I still like tennis, and playing singles is safer than a fast-reaction doubles game. Another good alternative is hitting against a tennis wall when I cannot find a partner. Using gym equipment is sometimes a challenge in selecting the weight or level of intensity. Also, since button labels on the machines are too small to read, I just hit a few and hope it works. I will say, yoga seems to be an easier choice for someone with low vision.

At a **movie theater**, I select a seat closer to the screen rather than one towards the back. I used to avoid libraries and bookstores, telling myself that this is no place for a blind person. I listened to a few books on tape and Audiobooks. However, I returned to reading books when I got the tools to read on my own.

Sad to say, watching **fireworks** is not nearly as enjoyable as it was when I had full sight. Maybe my brain is playing tricks on me, but every flash of light feels like I am damaging my retinas.

Current Problems

I've never considered myself to be a superb problem solver, although many other scientists excel at it. Maybe I was better at problem solving before my vision impairment. On the other hand, I'm sure I have to face and solve way more problems now.

Reading sheet music to play the cello or piano has been my biggest challenge and is one that has yet to be solved. Using a copy machine, I have enlarged sheet music to 200%, but it's still not large enough for me to read. I also have to keep the music stand about four feet away from my eyes, which is way too far to see.

In my younger years, I was excellent at sight reading. You could put a new piece of music in front of me, and I could play it pretty well the first time. Sadly, with low vision this ability is gone, so I've developed a strategy to memorize pieces one measure at a time. I hold the music page in my hand to look at it up close, then I place it down and play the notes I just read. I repeat this method, adding more notes as I go. Memorization was not something I had ever done in my cello lessons, but now it is the only way I am able to play.

When it comes to playing the piano, reading sheet music is challenging, but at least my eyes are closer to the music—only about one foot away. We have a player piano, with operating foot pedals that turn a roll. This roll has holes of different lengths and positions, indicating which key to depress and for how long. Although the player mechanism still works, the text on the rolls is fading and is usually too small for me to read.

Attitude of Persistence

Persistence is a key ingredient in coping with vision loss. When I encounter a vision obstacle, I tend to want to give up easily. My persistence (or lack thereof) also depends on whether I have encountered something similar before and what options are available to me. However, sometimes giving up is a step of self-preservation. With experience, I can estimate how long it will take me to do a particular task given certain tools. If it is substantially longer than the time it would take without a vision impairment, then I ask myself these questions: "Do I have the time available to complete this task and should I even attempt it? Should I ask another person to assist me or use a different device (for instance, better lighting)?" Negotiating these situations and making the decision of asking for help or going it alone is something I must continually do.

Summary

Although I have listed more than 20 tasks that are difficult to perform and the modifications I've had to make, I want to emphasize that there are still many things that I can do. I am very appreciative of that. In their work, Mogk and Mogk (2003) remind readers many times that macular degeneration patients should be resilient. Their message is, decide what you want to do and go do it. I feel like I am not as resilient as I'd like to be, but I've also found it helps to have something to look forward to in my schedule.

Although there were functional limitations to what I used to do easily, overall my quality of life did not fall dramatically. I learned new ways to do things and gave less emphasis to other tasks.

Chapter Eight
Fifteen Again

My nickname for this chapter is "Life Without a Driver's License."

After my vision diagnosis, I was fortunate that the changes in my vision and the deterioration of my visual acuity progressed slowly. After 11 years elapsed, my acuity changed from 20/30 to 20/100. With an acuity of 20/100, my doctor told me to stop driving. One might think that having a decade to prepare myself for this eventuality was plenty of time, but sadly, this change in driving status hit me hard. This time was almost as sorrowful as the month of my diagnosis.

Adapting to vision change was usually a slow process. It took me about a year to use a magnifier to read on a regular basis. However, when my optometrist informed me that my vision was too poor to drive one mile to my home and that I could no longer drive, that was a sudden and major life change. I knew that many patients with macular degeneration lose their driving privileges, but I approached that possibility with the hope that I would be one of the lucky ones who continued to drive. I definitely was in denial.

My Driving History
After my sixteenth birthday, I had about five or six hours of lessons from a driving school. I got my driver's license quickly. It was one of the first accomplishments I could claim as a teenager. I drove myself, and often my younger sister, to school,

music lessons, sports practices and work. At the time, I was fortunate to be living the typical teenage dream of having my own car. My parents fully paid for my first car, which was a 12-year-old dark green station wagon, truly a hand-me-down vehicle. We had a mutual understanding that I paid for gas and car insurance. The car broke down several times during my high school years, but I was a relatively responsible teenage driver. I just had one minor car accident: a bumper tap at low speed. As the car became less dependable, I switched to another used car, one that was only six years old.

After graduating from college, I traded in my second vehicle and bought a four-year-old car on my own. I received one speeding ticket at age 23. Driving was something that I took for granted. I made some long one-day road trips, including a few 750-mile drives from my mother's house to Tennessee. When I moved to Manhattan, I sold my car and was relieved to not have to worry about driving in the city. One reason was, I could not have afforded to park my vehicle in New York. Secondly, the New York public transportation system met my needs.

My driving story gets more interesting about five years after my vision diagnosis. My acuity had changed to 20/50, and I was driving my fourth car. I was visiting Atlanta in December and was having trouble driving in the dark. Downtown Atlanta was an unfamiliar place. I got horribly lost numerous times because I could not read the direction signs (the ones that instruct drivers which lane to take for certain destinations).

I visited an optometrist who explained that night blindness occurs with Stargardt disease. It made sense; I could not see well in the dark, especially in new places. This was my first realization that Stargardt disease was going to affect my lifestyle. One of my friends advised me to relocate and live near my workplace.

Returning to Tennessee, I tried to avoid driving at night because it was no longer safe. I began to adjust my daily schedule of activities. During the school year, I often worked in my office past sunset. That changed. I either had to leave my workplace before dark, or I had to move my home closer to work. I chose the latter option. I was living in Jackson, Tennessee, and the public transportation system consisted of only a few buses that did not appeal to me. I never learned the bus routes and, instead, found a house for sale within walking distance of work. After renting many apartments, I got a mortgage on my first house. I walked from my new home to my office on campus virtually every day. The decision to move certainly helped make my life more manageable. I no longer worried about getting to work. I ran errands on weekends during the daytime hours. However, I worried whether my disease would affect me doing my job.

My next job involved teaching and research at Allegheny College, located in Meadville, Pennsylvania, and at that time my acuity was about 20/50 in my better eye. My goal was to get a restricted driver's license for daytime driving. My experience with the Department of Motor Vehicles clerk was unpleasant, as many other people have told similar stories of clerks with nasty attitudes. I would imagine that it can be a hard job, as the clerk must tell people they are rejected for various reasons. At any rate, after I brought a note from my optometrist explaining my acuity and plans to drive in daytime only, I was able to get a Pennsylvania driver's license.

Change Happens When You Least Expect It
In the first two years after moving to Pennsylvania, I was a single woman who worked about 70 hours per week during each semester. My occupation was

the focus of my life; I loved teaching and was beginning to develop friendships. Meadville is a college and factory town, with the usual "town and gown" problems, where the townspeople and members of the college community do not get along. Aside from my neighbor and landlord, I didn't know anyone from town who was not connected to my employer. I rented a house one block from campus to make transportation to work easy. My only minor challenge was walking uphill on icy mornings.

The abrupt change in driving status occurred when I was 38 years old. My acuity had changed, as I had lost another line of vision on the Snellen eye chart. Patients, standing or sitting 20 feet away from the chart, read aloud the smallest line of letters or numbers that they can read. The lines are referred to as 20/x, with 20 indicating that they are 20 feet away from the chart. The "x" is a number, usually from 20 to 200 (25, 30, 40, 50, 70, 100). The second number refers to what a normally sighted individual, someone with 20/20 acuity, can see at a certain distance from the chart. For example, when a 20/20 individual is positioned 50 feet from the chart, he can see the 20/50 line of letters.

My acuity changed from 20/70 to 20/200, a change of two lines on the chart. A one-line change of acuity may not seem like a "big deal," but this loss caused a huge alteration in my life. In the Commonwealth of Pennsylvania, as in many other states, the minimum acuity deemed acceptable to drive was 20/70, so I was no longer qualified. It was in June of 2011 that my optometrist, Christopher Adsit, O.D., told me gently that I should not drive home. I don't recall my thoughts at that moment, but I know I sobbed in his office. After regaining my composure, I called a co-worker and asked if she could bring another colleague to drive me and my car home.

Dr. Adsit suggested that I schedule an appointment with a retina specialist to make sure that the acuity change was real and not temporary. About two weeks later, the retina specialist confirmed that my acuity was 20/150, a value still not able to drive legally. This doctor recommended that I contact a "blind office in Erie," which was either the Erie Sight Center or the Erie Office of Vocational Rehabilitation.

My previous words, "should not drive home," may require an explanation, as it has raised questions from many friends and family. If the legal minimum acuity is 20/70, then it is illegal for someone to drive with worse acuity, such as 20/100. I am one of those people who follow rules and laws. In many states, the legal minimum acuity is 20/40.

As a result of my rule-following personality, it didn't even occur to me to ignore my doctor's advice. I considered it my responsibility to stop driving immediately. If I had continued to drive with 20/100 acuity, I could have been involved in an accident. If so, my optometrist could have been liable for any damage that I caused. Worse yet, what if someone died as a result of my illegal driving? I'd feel terrible guilt and could face legal punishment. Of course, I believed I was a safe driver, but the risk of driving illegally was too great to take. Although I felt safe when driving in my town, the safety issue arose when I was driving on a highway or in an unfamiliar area.

Dustin Mitchell, O.D., another optometrist in Meadville, explained the perspective of the optometrist in this way in a note to me:

When I have a patient that does not meet the driving standards, I inform them at the end of the exam. It's just about as horrible for me, as an optometrist, to have that conversation as it is for the patient to hear it. It's taking a huge part of someone's life and independence away.

Eye doctors have several responsibilities at this stage. They must "document the conversation in the [patient's] chart and that the patient expressed understanding of the conversation that they are no longer legal to drive," Dr. Mitchell wrote to me. Then, they complete a form to document the patient is not currently meeting the vision standards for driving, and they state whether they recommend the person cease driving immediately or if the state should investigate, such as if the case is borderline. This form is submitted to the Department of Motor Vehicles in Pennsylvania, or the equivalent office in other states, immediately following the exam. Pennsylvania is referred to as a mandated reporter state.

Dr. Mitchell continued his explanation: "Most medical professionals are required to report it to the state when someone is no longer able to drive. If we fail to document anything and do not tell the patient to stop driving, we certainly could be held liable for what the patient did."

Initial Response to News

A reader might ask, "What was your emotional state after the news?" Well, I was distressed, an emotional wreck. I wrote about my feelings in a personal journal. When I re-read my journal entry from June 16, 2011, I thought it was worth sharing. June 16 was the day of my optometrist visit, the day my acuity officially changed to 20/200. My thoughts from that day are expressed in the following eight bullet points.

- This is horrible news, but I knew it was coming at some point in my life. I have had 11 years, one month and two weeks to prepare for it.
- I feel guilty for driving over the past month when my vision was so bad. But I didn't know it was **this** bad. I only felt unsafe one day, when I hit a dead animal on the highway because I saw it too late to avoid it.

- How could I drive with such bad vision? How could I not know?
- My friend Carolynn used this analogy for my vision change: it is like expecting a relative to die, and then that person dies. In my case, my vision died. The problem is, my life, as I know it, is gone. It's not the same as a person dying, for we all die at some point. Not all of us experience permanent vision loss.
- I feel like I lost a part of myself. The independent part of me that could drive to a restaurant or a park is dead.
- I wish I had a better support system in Meadville, but it's up to me to develop one.
- How do I tell Michael (my date last week)? What a lousy time to learn this information, at the very start of a relationship! How am I ever going to date someone if I can't leave Meadville? I told Michael that the doctor had given me "bummer news."
- Thank goodness I'm not in Atlanta now, as I would be worrying about how to get rides and how to get back to Pennsylvania.

I shared the news of my vision status with a few friends and family members. Not everyone answered the phone, and "I felt like the world had deserted me." I told the research student working with me that summer, who was quite empathetic. I was fortunate to have a job that I could do. I threw myself into my work. I told my two closest friends in Tennessee, and my friend Peggy from The Foundation Fighting Blindness. I was relieved that my mother took on the burden of telling most of our relatives. It was so hard emotionally to tell people that I could no longer drive. My vision loss felt like a heavy weight.

Coping and Grief
The stages of grief were ever-present. Besides those

stages, I experienced irritability, numbness and apathy. I craved routine; working in my office allowed for a distraction from my sadness and anxiety.

When I was diagnosed with Stargardt disease, I had a strong support system in Nashville. When I lost my driver's license, sadly, my support system was puny. The local friends I had developed were acquaintances, not yet trustworthy. Playing music on the cello was comforting, as some of my favorite pieces are sorrowful. I went to the campus minister to discuss my faith. I considered volunteering in the community by helping others, so I could temporarily forget my own problems.

Life without Driving

I had driven for 22 years. During the three years when I lived in Manhattan, although I couldn't afford to keep a car, at least I still had a driver's license. In my adult life, I had taken driving for granted. The loss of my driving privileges was the most difficult adjustment I had to make; it was harder than the loss of a love relationship. I equated adulthood with driving, and I believed that not driving made me less of a person. I felt like I was 15 years old again, waiting for a ride from my mother to a music lesson or from the medical center where I volunteered. Since she was often late to pick me up, I spent what seemed like a lot of time waiting.

In the first month after I stopped driving, my mother visited, and we stocked my cupboards with food. After she left, I inevitably ran out of milk and was very sad. I was in denial. I seemed unable to take any steps to get more milk. I didn't want to ask my colleagues for a ride to the grocery store. However, during one of my weak moments, I cried in front of someone I barely knew, and she offered to take me. I was an emotional mess!

I wondered, "How will I tell my co-workers?" Allegheny College was a small institution with about

300 employees, and I knew almost half of them. I asked my department chairperson to notify my co-workers, the 25 people who worked in the same building. Since it was July and many folks were on vacation, she sent a blanket email to everyone informing them of my vision change and that I was seeking car rides. Unfortunately, in terms of transportation assistance, this strategy backfired.

In response to the email request to my 25 immediate co-workers, I received one email reply and two in-person offers for rides. One woman offered to take me with her on errands on Saturdays at 8 a.m., although the timing and store were not ideal. Sometimes, I accepted her standing offer. I felt that the phrase "beggars can't be choosers" applied to me. Another co-worker offered me a ride from a meeting when it was snowing. The rest of my colleagues didn't offer to help at all.

I walked to the grocery store twice per week. Carrying two bags of groceries up a steep hill was not appealing to me, but did I have any other options? By the time classes resumed in August, no one was offering me rides to the grocery store. I wrote, "The world goes on, not thinking of my needs."

I hated asking for rides. The worst part was that my closest friends lived far away in another state. Most of my co-workers were acquaintances, not friends I could rely upon. I was reticent to ask them for rides, and when I did, I learned that some of them were not reliable. Whenever anyone canceled, I was incredibly disappointed. I felt guilty asking for rides. In 2011, my life in Meadville was quite sheltered; my world was isolated, and my colleagues were very busy. It seemed that no one had free time to do me a favor. This did not help my self-esteem or relationship-building skills, as I felt I was a burden to others.

In the first six months of not driving, I valued everyone who gave me a ride. I developed a pattern of asking for rides from friends who worked outside my department. It felt too much of an obligation to ask a co-worker. I began to expect less from my co-workers; they just did not understand my situation and I was tired of begging for rides. I think the reason I expected my co-workers to assist me was because at my previous employer, Lambuth University, I had many friends who worked with me. I had about five friends who would have done almost anything for me. Say what you will about the South and western Tennessee, but the people there are mighty friendly. Tennessee got the nickname of the Volunteer State for its military recruits, but volunteerism is a regular habit.

At the time, I lived one block from where I worked, and I usually walked to work daily. While this is certainly convenient, the negative part was that I felt like I was always working and could never leave my workplace. Without a driver's license, if I wanted to go anywhere except the college, I needed to pay for transportation.

With all of these changes in 2011 due to not driving, I did a few other things in my personal life. According to my journal, I threw myself into my work and exercised more regularly than I had ever done before. I tried to make more social plans, which was semi-successful. I also saw a counselor regularly.

Attitude Change

The first step in accepting my non-driving status was adjusting my attitude about asking for help. For one reason, there were people who wanted to help me; they just didn't know how to offer. I would walk to the garage and check on my car, something I never did when I was allowed to drive. I regularly felt depressed when I saw my car sitting in the garage. It was such an odd feeling for me because I had never had any feelings for my car. I had depended on my vehicle, paid for the routine maintenance, and took it for granted. Finally, one friend bought my ten-year-old car and I stopped obsessing about it.

About a year after I stopped driving, I relinquished my driver's license and converted it to an identification card. This was not so emotionally wrenching, mainly because I had given myself time to grieve the loss.

One of the consequences of living within walking distance of my employment was that I felt like I was always working. I literally could not get away from campus without assistance. There were several winters when I spent at least eight weeks within a ten-mile radius of my house and work (Crawford County). This is what I consider the worst part of not driving: the lack of variety in my life. As Georgina Kleege (1999, 29) notes, "Your freedom is seriously restricted if you can't drive."

Jennifer Rothschild was diagnosed with retinitis pigmentosa at age 15 and was never allowed to get a driver's license. Since she cannot drive, she often experiences delayed gratification and waits for some personal items. "I have to wait until someone else is heading to the store. I get my needs and desires met according to someone else's schedule, rarely my own" (Rothschild 2002, 199). Accepting that we are not the decision makers is not easy.

Advice to Non-drivers
When an adult stops driving, there are a few things to consider:

1. Walking may become a more frequent part of your life out of necessity. Find one or two pairs of walking shoes and wear weather-appropriate clothing.

2. Find a mode of transportation that suits you. If available, learn the schedule of that transportation and keep a copy of it with you, or memorize it.

3. Find a local organization that offers low-price transportation. In Pennsylvania, a non-profit group called Keystone Blind Association has the mission of transporting visually-impaired residents to medical appointments. Some organizations ask for a minimal fee, while others have a fee depending on the ride distance.

4. Prioritize your errands. I became a more organized person because I could not depend on others to take me to multiple locations. I learned that some stores fit more than one category. Why should I go to a department store, a pharmacy and a grocery store, if one retail store meets all three needs? I began to shop more often at Walmart and Target because I could find more items at a single store.

Getting groceries was probably my biggest weekly challenge. I had to plan ahead. If I ran out of an item, I could not easily "run to the store." This was especially true if I were making dinner and the buses stopped running in the evening. Would it be safe for me to walk home from the grocery store in the dark?

5. Use "Plan G" for getting a ride. This was advice from a speaker at an FFB-sponsored VISIONS conference. Sometimes the first person you ask for a ride (Plan A) is not available, and the second person (Plan B) is also not available. On rare occasions, you may need Plans C to F, all the way to Plan G. Once, in July 2014, I experienced Plan G because my cell phone died. I asked six people for a ride to and from a haircut appointment; one was able to drop me off, but all were busy at the time of my return. I literally could not find a ride. So, I walked three miles from the salon to my home. Unfortunately, the first mile was on a dangerous road with no sidewalks. Desperate times call for desperate measures.

Final Observations

For about two years after I stopped driving, I received phone calls from my insurance company, asking me why I had canceled my car insurance policy. I guess my reason was not a common one. I cried every time they called. It bothered me so much that I called my local insurance agent to explain. He apologized on behalf of the company. I asked if he could instruct the home office not to call me again. The message took years to get through, and I continued to receive calls.

Being independent and controlling my transportation were such important parts of my adult life. I don't understand people who choose not to drive, despite being healthy, capable of driving and financially able to afford a vehicle. Of course, I'm not referring to people with access to good public transportation systems like New York City, Washington, D.C. and Chicago. Do they like being dependent on someone for travel? For me personally, driving has always been a huge advantage in daily independent living.

Chapter Nine
The Lows of Public Transportation

Transportation is a major issue for any patient with vision loss and particularly for those with low vision. The Foundation Fighting Blindness recommends living in cities with public transportation. The problem, of course, is that my career field has a limited number of jobs. In some years, there might be ten advertised positions for physiologists at teaching colleges in the United States, but only a few of them are "good fits." Adding a requirement of "must have good public transportation" on top of that definitely can be a deal breaker.

In Manhattan, I walked about ten blocks from my apartment to my job at a medical campus. On weekends, I took the A train on the Metro Transit Authority (MTA) when I was socializing, attending church and educating myself on urban culture. I rarely took the bus, except when I was crossing Central Park.

Transportation in Meadville
In Meadville, population 13,388 (in 2010), a friend of a friend explained the Crawford (County) Area Transportation Authority (CATA) system to me. There were three bus routes. The Red line was the one that went past campus and came closest to my residence. It repeated its loop every hour from 8 a.m. to 8 p.m. and ran Monday through Saturday; there was no service on Sundays. We made a Sat-

urday appointment to take the bus together and I learned how to request a stop. The bus was truly helpful in meeting many of my weekly transportation needs. After this introduction, I took it two or three times per week and did not have to ask for as many rides.

Early on, I had mixed feelings about the CATA bus. For one thing, I needed the bus but hated my dependency. For a few months, I would cry while waiting for the bus. I resented being the youngest person on the bus; I felt like I did not belong there. Eventually, I accepted my fate. The purpose of the bus was for non-drivers to get out of their houses. I was tired of walking the entire distance from home to my destination, so walking to and from the bus stops saved my feet from soreness. I certainly couldn't complain about the low price ($1, then $1.25) for a ride. Sometimes I was the only passenger and spoke with the driver.

The Red line and I had issues over the years. I recall numerous occasions when I was waiting for the bus. It either did not come or went past me without stopping. At least once, the driver yelled at me for not waving at him. Apparently, most passengers who are car-less are not blind like me. Eventually, I explained to this driver that I had poor vision; if I could see well enough to identify the bus from a distance, I would be driving myself. In my July 2013 journal, I noted that in one very hot week, I walked from my home to downtown four times. I had intended to take the bus, but either the bus was not running or did not stop to pick me up.

Two years later, CATA Operations decided to establish official bus stops marked by signs, solving this problem. It was rare for a bus driver to not stop when I was waiting at an official bus stop, but it was frustrating when it did happen. On several occasions, the bus route changed without notice.

Sometimes it was running normally in the morning but suddenly altered in the afternoon. This was particularly irksome to me. At those times, I had three options. I could call CATA headquarters to ask if something happened to the bus. I could wait an hour for the next one. Or I could walk the whole distance. Unfortunately, if the bus needed repair, there was no way to inform potential passengers that the bus was not running. I had the impression that there were no spare buses to take over when one stopped working. Based on my five years of experience, I would rate the CATA bus Red route with a B- for dependability.

Another challenge for bus passengers is that some networks have restrictions on how many bags a passenger can bring aboard. CATA's rules are that the passenger's bags must either fit on the lap or at the feet; bags cannot block the aisle. Basically, large items cannot be brought onto the bus, even if they can be easily carried. This rule really impacts those who rely on the bus as their only means of transportation. One time I observed a driver deny a passenger entrance because she wanted to carry a bulky item on board. This left her hiring a taxi instead of paying for a bus ride.

One last point related to public transportation: I currently live in a county where there is no public transportation whatsoever. It qualifies as a rural county, but my village is located five miles from two towns that do have bus service. This is a trade-off for my village; most roads have sidewalks on both sides of the street, but there is no public transportation.

Keystone Blind Association

My mother discovered the local chapter of Keystone Blind Association (KBA) in Crawford County. The closest main office was located in Sharon, Pennsylvania (now in Hermitage). KBA provided rides to doctor's appointments in and near Meadville, as well as eye doctor appointments in Erie (50 minutes away) or Pittsburgh (more than 90 minutes away).

The KBA drivers accompanied the clients to the waiting room and even helped to complete medical forms, filling out what the patients told them about their medical history. These forms were never in large print. I often wondered why health care providers, especially those who treat elderly patients, did not provide them. This is yet another way that visually-impaired people must adapt.

Clients also can use KBA services for things like rides to the grocery store or Walmart. These regular trips were offered on weekdays, which suited clients who were retired, disabled or unemployed. I was the only client who held a full-time job, so I was unable to use this option due to my teaching duties. Finding a ride to my haircut appointments was my biggest challenge since there was no public transportation to that area.

The KBA organization offered more than I have described. The administrative director of the Crawford County office, Bob George, was a friendly man who tried to raise the morale of his clients. Whenever one called the KBA answering service, there was a positive, uplifting daily message that Bob selected. He understood that his blind clients experience loneliness. I wondered if living in a rural area, such as Crawford County, worsened that feeling for me.

Through KBA I met people in the county who were not connected to my employer, people who were like me and had vision disorders. I was indeed the youngest adult to use their services and was told by several optometrists that I was the only Stargardt patient in the county.

Taxi Service
A reader might ask, "Why didn't you use a taxi service or Uber for rides?" Well, I tried this option a

few years after I stopped driving. To avoid walking downtown in a blizzard, I called the only taxi service in Meadville. The dispatcher told me that all of the taxis were booked for the entire day. How disappointing! A few weeks later, I called again and got the same answer. Although taxis might be useful in certain places, the taxi service in Meadville was sadly lacking. When I lived in Manhattan, I considered taking a taxi as a special occasion. They were expensive relative to the subway and bus, and sometimes the New York City cab drivers were not very nice.

The services of Uber and Lyft are certainly improvements. Unfortunately, for the five years I lived in Meadville without a driver's license, there was only one Uber driver by the fifth year. Frankly, that wasn't much help, and for the occasions when I was seeking a ride, the local Uber driver wasn't even working. This was discernible from the application output, indicating that the closest available driver was 30 minutes away. Although both of these companies offer transportation options for many people, they were not dependable or accessible where I lived. There is a lesson to learn here: people who want rides should live in densely populated areas instead of a rural county.

The other problem with Lyft and Uber is the small text of their mobile applications. The text cannot be enlarged on the devices at my disposal. This was also frustrating, as I probably would make use of their services more often if I were able to read the text. In its current state, my track record of successful rides is three out of six attempts. If I cannot read the description of the vehicle to expect or the name of the driver, it becomes a challenge to be able to find the vehicle and the driver when the ride arrives. This is an even bigger problem in inclement weather;

most potential passengers would prefer to wait indoors for the ride, but doing so often makes it harder to see an approaching vehicle. Maybe being able to speak with the driver in advance, to explain that I'm not able to see cars clearly, would help. Lastly, some locations or businesses do not allow a car to park and wait. I found that using these applications with low vision can be more trouble than it is worth.

Greyhound Buses

When I stopped driving, I was unwilling to stop traveling, but my savings account was small. Some of my destinations were achievable by plane, while others were accessible by road. I investigated the Greyhound bus schedule (www.greyhound.com) and made several reservations.

My Greyhound travels have taken me from Meadville, Pennsylvania, to Harrisburg, New York City, Washington, D.C., Cleveland and Akron. Switching buses occurred in either Pittsburgh or Erie stations. I also have taken it from Jackson, Tennessee, to Atlanta, Georgia, through Nashville and Chattanooga. Some of that long travel was very smooth, especially when I didn't have to change buses.

My main complaint was the limitations in timing options. To travel from Meadville to Akron, it was a two-hour direct drive. By bus the whole trip took six hours and cost about $40. I took a southbound bus to Pittsburgh with a two-hour layover at the station, then switched to a bus heading west to Youngstown and Akron.

Additional delays are never fun. A regular rider becomes accustomed to delays. I considered it a successful trip if the bus arrived within 30 minutes of its expected arrival time. Perhaps that is similar in air travel. While in bus stations, I have been approached by beggars, people just released from prison (to use my cell phone), and some par-ent-less children.

Speaking of other riders, people with prominent tattoos are more likely to sit next to me on a bus than on a train or plane. Buses are usually noisi-er than trains or planes. Bus riders are advised to bring a listening device with a charger. However, on a bus, passengers can interact more with the driver, as opposed to a pilot or train conductor (for good or bad). Not every driver was in a good mood, and a bus with no air conditioning in the summer can be downright ugly!

Another disadvantage of riding a bus a long dis-tance is the feeling of responding to a cattle call. Some people complain about this on airplanes, but at least when you board a plane, the attendant (as well as the ticket clerk and Transportation Securi-ty Agent) looks at your name and identification. On a Greyhound bus, passengers are nameless. When switching buses, one needs to be within hearing range of the gate. Announcements of departure or changes such as a different gate or a delay may be oral rather than visual. At airports, sometimes the airline pages passengers personally before the flight takes off. For a bus ride, there is no such personal calling. The next bus headed in that di-rection could be as little as 4 hours later or as long as 24 hours later.

Amtrak Trains
For visually-impaired travelers, trains are a good option. The signage is generally clear and many announcements are made audibly. It is an interme-diate experience—more personal than Greyhound but less luxurious than an airplane trip. My favor-ite route was the four-hour Keystone route, cost-ing about $50. It ran from Harrisburg to New York, Penn Station, with 13 local stops from the capital to Philadelphia, and then a few stops in New Jer-

sey. Plus, there were about six Keystone trains per day ranging from departures in morning to early evening, adding to convenience.

My main complaint about Amtrak (www.amtrak.com) is coverage. Amtrak does not go to enough cities or offer enough daily routes. The phrase "can't get there from here" applies to a number of destinations. For instance, to go from Pittsburgh to Cleveland, one must first go to Chicago or New York, neither of which is convenient. Simply put, you can't go from certain cities to others without having to change several times or have a long layover.

When All Else Fails, Walk

Walking is my go-to option when the weather is tolerable. Whether I am in an airport or in a new city, life often involves asking for directions. My pet peeve is when someone says, "You can't miss it." I have to stifle my response of "Oh yeah? I bet I can." Ryan Knighton notes in his book, *Cockeyed* (2006, 103), that the words "this," "that" and "there" are too vague to be helpful to blind people. "Over there" and "that way" are only useful if one can see the direction that someone is indicating with his or her hands or head. A much better answer would be, for example, "50 feet to your right."

Chapter Ten
Adjustments in Social Life

The social aspect of vision loss is often overlooked, but it is quite important. An inability to see clearly impacts conversations and many interactions with others. I first appreciated this when Hull (1990, 29) commented, "The whole structure of our ordinary everyday conversation presupposes a sighted world." Think how often we use visual terms in our conversation, even when it is not needed.

For almost a decade, I was very sensitive to over-using the words "see," "sight" and "vision" in conversations. I avoided the common responses like "See ya later" and "Looking forward to it." After I received a promotion that had been delayed for two years, it really upset me when the female dean told me, "It was an oversight," when describing her mistake over the delay. Her error was small; she failed to change my rank from Visiting Assistant Professor to Assistant Professor (only in academia would that title matter). But how could she have used the word "oversight" to a blind person? At some point I realized that I am just one person against the world. Will I be able to change society's use of these words? Of course not! All I am capable of is selecting my own vocabulary. As a visually-challenged person, telling people that I am sensitive to using words about vision is like announcing that I am not comfortable with my blindness. For nearly a decade, that was my situation.

As a result, this sensitivity sent a message to others to avoid me socially.

What I Say about My Vision to Others

When I meet strangers, I must decide whether they need to know anything about my vision. There are plenty of situations where it is best to disclose my vision status early on. One of those situations is at a doctor's office. I usually say something rather general like, "I have a visual impairment," rather than specifying macular degeneration or Stargardt disease. Unless the doctor studies eyes, the staff and the doctor will probably not be familiar with Stargardt disease. The specifics do not matter to most people.

In my 30s, one of the lines I used was, "I have the eyes of an 80-year-old." This is confusing to people because there are a few 80-year-olds who have rather good vision. Unless I am in a young audience, that line is not effective.

In her book *Lessons I Learned in the Dark* (2002), Jennifer Rothschild shares that it is hard to describe her vision to people on a daily basis. It was not obvious to others that she could not see. Her blindness due to retinitis pigmentosa could be hidden "behind a façade that made me feel 'normal'" (137). Macular degeneration patients have a similar issue. We do not look like we cannot see.

Two Common Questions

There are two questions that I am frequently asked about my vision. First is, "What does it feel like to have macular degeneration?" My snarky answer is, "Duh, close your eyes." I get the question's point, though. It is not easy to put into words what central vision loss is like, how I can see some things but not others. Try to imagine walking into a store with a sign on the wall and not being able to read it. Sometimes I feel like I am in a foreign land where another language is spoken. Maybe blindness is like any chronic health problem. On a daily basis, it can be annoying because it affects certain aspects of living.

Second is, "How do you manage life with a visual impairment?" I could ask the person a similar question: "How do **you** manage your life with the burdens and health issues that you have accrued?" I suspect what the curious really are wondering is something like, "How do you complete certain life activities if you can't see?" Naturally, not everything is obvious, and there is a lot to learn about being blind. Chapter Thirteen tackles some of these daily challenges.

There is another way to approach this question. If the person means, "How do you get through life?" My short answer is, "Find something that makes you want to get out of bed each morning." Then re-read Chapter Two.

Social Situations and Macular Degeneration

With central vision loss, two of the most frustrating aspects about social interactions are not being able to recognize faces and not seeing people's expressions. In large group settings, like a party, I would love to be able to recognize someone from ten feet away or more. With 20/110 acuity, this is not possible. I am lucky if I can recognize my friend at that distance. Asking, "Have we met before?" or re-introducing myself is sometimes socially acceptable.

When entering a room with a lot of sunlight, I select a seat with my back to the sun. At one department retreat, I went to lunch and returned to find that my previous seat had been claimed by a co-worker. I tried to politely explain, in front of the entire department, why it was necessary for me to sit in the seat facing away from the bright sun. If I could have a do-over, I would approach the sitter, ask to speak privately away from the others, and make my request one-on-one.

Dating

Dating with a visual impairment adds an extra level of complication. Usually one is already nervous, wondering if the date will like him or her or not. Add to this my question of "When should I disclose my visual impairment?" Is the right time when speaking on the phone, when planning a date or when meeting face to face? Should it be a casual mention in conversation or a deal-breaker issue?

When my vision was slightly impaired, say an acuity of 20/40, I usually waited to disclose this information to a date—unless a situation arose in which I could not hide it. For instance, if we went to a darkened restaurant for a first date, in what the food industry calls "mood lighting," then I could not read the menu. Is there a polite way of telling someone that you cannot read in low light settings? I found this mildly awkward.

As my vision worsened, I felt more vulnerable on dates, as I had to ask for transportation to and from the event. Particularly in the year after I stopped driving, I lacked confidence and had to adjust to my changing body. In regards to using magnifiers at restaurants, I will share one pathetic story. One of my dates laughed at me when I showed him my hand-held magnifier. While I was proud of myself for bringing the magnifier with me to read the menu by myself, he had a different view. Regardless of whether he was laughing at me or at the situation, he was not sensitive. This was a clear sign that not everyone is capable of a relationship with a blind person. In retrospect, I have asked myself whether this uncomfortable situation could have been avoided.

In the case of dating the man who became my husband, our dating life was nothing to brag about.

I was awkward when I discussed my vision and other topics. But when Donald was in college, one of his favorite courses was taught by a professor who was blind since childhood. My belief is that because he had a positive experience with a blind person in authority, Donald was not uncomfortable to enter a dating relationship with someone with a visual impairment. Thank goodness that he was able to overcome my awkwardness and see the real person inside.

Nonverbal Communication
In many social and work environments, nonverbal communication is critical. It includes gestures, facial expressions, eye contact, distance between two people, body language, posture, tone of voice and touch, according to Wikipedia. Many of these features are visual, leaving the blind person at a disadvantage during conversations. I don't know how to fix this issue, but I definitely suffered the negative effects of not being able to read the nonverbal cues of the people I worked with. I never intend to be rude or dismissive, but some people perceive me in this way. Once I became aware of this misperception, I took steps to correct it. One way to do so was to explain it to my students on the first day of class. Sadly, I was unable to explain this to my supervisors when my vision first deteriorated. There are claims that nonverbal communication contributes 60 to 70% to a conversation, says Wikipedia. If this is true, blind people might be missing a big part of everyday interactions.

Social Isolation and Blind Organizations
"One of the most difficult aspects of blindness is the way it tends to make you passive in getting to know people" (Hull 1990, 97). Even with macular degeneration, there is social marginalization and passivity. Kals and Lauerman (2000, 81) noted that

"the most frustrating effect of the disease may be isolation and loneliness." One doctor suspects that one-third of her AMD patients are depressed and "feel helpless and angry." Kals and Lauerman (2000, 81) advised, "Finally, if a friend or loved one suffers from AMD, be patient and understanding." With all of the challenges in daily living associated with macular degeneration, it is comforting when my friends and co-workers accept me and treat me like everyone else. I did not want to be identified as "the blind person," for I was the only one, and isolation means social rejection.

Talking with other visually-impaired or blind people breaks down social isolation. There is a time period of processing for the patient, adapting to vision loss. Where does one find visually-impaired people? Many communities have them and the main keyword is "blind." In Nashville, there was the group Prevent Blindness as well as the Tennessee Council for the Blind. I was unaware of these groups when I lived there. In Meadville, the local group was Keystone Blind Association (KBA). In Northeast Ohio, there are Blind Centers in Akron, Canton and Cleveland. The Akron Blind Center offers about 20 classes to their members, ranging from lessons in Braille, computer technology, crafts and Bible trivia.

As Bob George of KBA explained to me,

Socialization is a critical part of why KBA exists. Many visually impaired people don't have the opportunity to socialize, so being able to meet in a group of six or eight and commiserate is almost magical. They speak in their own lingo, and they understand what frustration the others are expressing because they are all visually impaired.

Benefits of Macular Degeneration

Though it may seem surprising, my work life has actually improved in several ways because of my vision loss. When I was a college student, I was a rather non-forgiving tutor. I thought that if you could not learn the material as quickly as I could, it meant that you were less intelligent. This was a naïve attitude. Thankfully, my perspective on learning has changed dramatically after encountering my own adversity. By the time I began teaching, I was willing to approach my students using different methods to get my point across. I was more understanding of those with learning difficulties, and my empathy level rose.

I rarely encountered students with vision loss. The one student with Stargardt disease in my introductory biology class changed her major to psychology. She was repeating the course because, in the previous semester, the professor did not post class materials in advance. Having the class materials to review before class is crucial; it takes me so long to read content that I would miss many points made in a lecture when I did not have access to it earlier.

I understand why the student changed her major, and it probably was the right decision. There are some biology professors, and probably chemistry and physics professors as well, who are not willing to adjust their courses to accommodate a blind student. It is an attitude in which the burden of learning is placed entirely on the student. "If you can't find a way to learn this material, you won't be successful later, so why should I help you now?"

Pet Peeve about Oral Presentations

Having macular degeneration has made me appreciate oral presentations more than I had before. Obviously preparing a presentation involves organizing slides and applying the Goldilocks rule to get the amount of text "just right." Equally important are the words the speaker uses. Unless I sit in the front row, I can't read the content of the slides and so am focused more on what speakers say. It is the only part of a presentation that I can access. When I teach, I consider that my students have different learning styles; some prefer visual while others learn by listening. For both of these types, my slides and oratory must be top-notch. I ask myself, "If a member of the audience is only able to hear me and not see the slide, what information is critical?"

In my experience, many speakers let the slides do the majority of their presentation (speak for them), and their spoken words are unclear. I agree with Georgina Kleege (2015) when she commented that "PowerPoint is like assistive technology for the sighted," and they spend less time preparing what they will say to a visual audience. There are so many examples of academics making visual presentations and forgetting their audience.

My number one pet peeve during presentations is the phrase, "As you can see," because it stigmatizes the audience. First, it is a useless phrase. Can you get your point across without using it? How does it help the listener understand? I used to feel insulted by this line because the speaker was assuming that everyone in the audience was fully sighted. Second, what if the listener is blind or cannot see the screen clearly or where the speaker is indicating? What if one can see the image but does not know what he or she is looking at? This can give a negative impression to audience members. Then it raises audience anxiety, wondering, "What am I missing? Am I too dumb to understand this?"

If the speaker is interested in being understood and in truly communicating effectively, then this situation can easily be addressed. I suggest saying, for example, "The figure on the left shows ... " followed by a descriptive sentence indicating what is on the slide. This helps both the sighted and unsighted audience members. "This figure shows" does not insult the listener, and a laser pointer is not necessary. Some speakers want the audience to do the mental work of drawing conclusions from the results, but the point of a presentation is to share information. I believe it is best to simply make your points and then discuss them, using a respectful manner to communicate.

My favorite story of this problem was at a seminar promoting vision research, sponsored by the Foundation Fighting Blindness. Many audience members had a vision disease. The speaker pointed at confocal microscope images and said, "as you can see," multiple times. I considered raising my hand and telling her it was offensive to assume that we could see what she was pointing at. I was one of the few scientists in the room and even I was struggling to understand. Perhaps a helpful analogy is the expectant couple asking the ultrasound technician or healthcare professional to determine if the fetus is male or female. How many pregnant women have looked at the sonogram and wondered if that speck was a penis? The professional should clearly point on the screen to the area for genitalia and say, "This is how I know it's a boy."

Chapter Eleven
Employment Issues and Adjustments

As a gradual and progressive disease, macular degeneration affects one's career in various ways. However, if the patient is retired when visual symptoms begin to appear, this chapter may not be relevant.

Career Thoughts

When I was diagnosed with Stargardt disease, I was 27 years old. In terms of my future career path, I sought advice from my mentor, dissertation committee members and the chairman of my department. I asked, "What type of career could I have in science if I lost my vision? What would I be able to do?" Unfortunately, they didn't have any answers.

I wondered if my previous five years of training would turn out to have been a waste of time. We agreed that my short-term focus should be on completing and defending my dissertation and getting a degree. My next goal would be to investigate career options. I decided upon a post-doctoral fellowship in the field of vitamin A and vision, allowing me to learn more about my disease through my work.

I began research on vitamin A at Columbia University and soon found I needed an assistant—a lab technician—to run some biochemical tests. I couldn't see well enough to do them myself. I made a schedule for when I wanted the technician to

work with me, and experiments got done in a timely manner. I had no complaints about getting assistance for my work.

On the surface, my work appeared to be successful and supported. However, a journal entry from
November 2001 indicates that things were not so
rosy. After a long day of data collection, one of my
research mentors shouted at me, "If you can't see,
get out of science!" About an hour later, he did offer a semi-apology. This was my first experience
of anti-blindness sentiment at work.

Job Interviews

There were two pressing questions related to job
interviews and blindness. The first was, "What
should I **say** at a job interview about my vision?"
The second was, "What should I **avoid** mention-
ing about my vision?" I wondered whether to inform the interviewers about my potential disability. This term, "potential disability," is interesting:
does anyone truly know in advance when he or she
will achieve a disabled state? Disabling accidents
can happen to anyone at any time, and progressive
diseases rarely follow a predictive, timely format.

The consistent advice I received was to not disclose any information about my vision, for two
reasons. First, this information could be used to
discriminate against hiring me. Second, job performance is not directly tied to vision. Keeping
my personal medical information secret was my
main goal.

I applied for many jobs in academia, with the primary selection factors being academic field (physiology), geographic location (east of the Mississippi
River), and type of institution (teaching-focused).
Following the advice to not disclose my potential
disability, I carefully constructed my written application materials so that there was no mention of
blindness. Some applications involve checking box-

es for ethnicity, sex, disability and veteran status. When my vision worsened, I dutifully checked the disabled box. This information is reported to the Employment or Human Resources office and not shared with the search committee. In the academic hiring process, the first selection is based entirely on the written application, consisting of cover letter, curriculum vitae (CV, an academic résumé), teaching philosophy, research statement and reference letters.

A second interview in academia is done by phone or on-campus. When I was selected for an interview, sometimes I would hide my vision status, and other times I would disclose it during the second interview. As my disease progressed, I became more comfortable discussing my vision status.

Depending on the interview requirements, I sometimes needed to disclose my visual challenges to the person who planned my itinerary. For instance, if the interview involved reading, then it would be helpful to request printing reading materials in 14 point. I learned this lesson the hard way: during one on-campus interview, the committee gave me a printed list of questions in 10 point, and the only way I could read them was with a hand-held magnifier. Although I do not have mobility issues, I know some people with peripheral vision loss who request, in advance, a sighted guide for a campus tour.

One of my sources of job interview advice was the Blind Academics listserv, a group bulletin board via email that shares common problems and solutions experienced by its members. An academic job search has multiple hurdles, and blind job candidates find unique ways to tackle some obstacles. One posting by Angela Frederick in 2017 inspired me. She shared a letter she wrote to a school (I have omitted its name) prior to a campus interview:

As my visit is approaching, I want to share with you and the other members of the search committee that I am blind. I have been losing my eyesight slowly as the result of an eye disease called Retinitis Pigmentosa. I have lost my remaining vision while in graduate school.

I take a very practical approach to my disability. I view blindness, not as a tragedy or a sensitive topic to be avoided, but as a nuisance that can be managed effectively through alternative techniques and a little innovation.

I expect that you and the other committee members will have many questions about how I manage my work, and I am happy to answer all of your inquiries. I always say that I would rather answer 100 questions about my blindness than experience the consequences of one negative assumption made about my competence.

I would likely need just one or two accommodations in order to perform effectively at … Regarding the campus visit … If it is comfortable for everyone, I would prefer to take your arm as I walk with you during my visit so that I can concentrate on getting to know all of you and the college. But, I wanted you to know that assistance with mobility is not an accommodation I would need were I to be offered and accept the position. … Other than this, there aren't any accommodations I will need during my visit.

I aspire to demonstrate the perspective of her second paragraph.

Upon reflection after various job searches, I have realized that hiding my disability does not benefit me. If my potential co-workers have an issue with blindness, it is better to clear up any confusion at the outset. However, if blindness is a sticking point, then this is probably an indication that I would not enjoy working there. Although this situation could rise to the level of illegal job discrimination, I think proving that can be tricky. Fortunately, the job market today is more open-minded than it used to be.

For one position, I disclosed my vision status in an email two weeks before the scheduled on-campus interview. One week later, I was told that the entire search was canceled. Did the school cancel my interview because of my disability? I'll never know. Is it worth my time to worry about this possibility? Nope.

Disclosing My Vision Status to Students

Early in my teaching career, I hid my vision problem from students. I believed that they would be more likely to cheat if they knew I had a weakness. I wondered, "How could I report cheating if I could not see students clearly?" My first institution, Lambuth University in Jackson, Tennessee, did not have an official honor code, and faculty members routinely shared stories of ways that students tried to cheat in their classes.

At my next school, the assistant dean encouraged me to tell students more about my vision. He was right; the students were very receptive when I told them that I had a form of macular degeneration and that the class would run differently in a few ways. For instance, in order to get my attention in class, students may need to wave their hands, as I can easily detect movement but might miss an unmoving raised hand. For writing assignments, I asked them to write legibly with large letters or use 14-point type. They adjusted so well to these minor changes that many students forgot I was blind. I had to remind them that I could not read the 12-point text on their exams, when a student would point to a question. I had been printing my lecture notes in 14 point since 2006.

The main adjustment in my teaching due to vision changes related to grading. If a student's handwriting was difficult to read, I asked that student to type his or her answers instead. For the cardio-vascular unit exam (Animal Physiology), I designed an oral exam with multiple essay questions. I gave students ten potential essay questions about one week in advance. They were supposed to prepare answers to all of the questions. At the time of the exam, each student would draw two numbers, and they would answer those two questions. If they did not address something on my grading rubric, I could ask them for clarification (such as, "Can you tell me anything about diastolic pressure?"). They usually gave answers in front of three other students in a shared learning experience, but I gave them the option of doing it one-on-one with me as well. Being able to answer orally indicated how well they knew the material, and it saved me hours of reading their written answers.

Office Frustrations
A frequent problem for me was the photocopier. I repeatedly selected the wrong person's name (be-cause the text was too small to read my name clearly) and sent a scan unintentionally to a co-worker. I got so tired of this mistake and hav-ing to apologize for not being able to see my own name. My solution was to stop being embarrassed about it and just bring a magnifier with me when using the copier.

Asking for Accommodations
I have had three academic jobs since my vision worsened and have asked for accommodations in different ways. Early on, at Lambuth University, I didn't know how to ask for help, and the school had a shoestring budget. In December of 2005, I spoke with the head of our school about getting a student helper to grade homework and quizzes, as there was much grading in my 13-credit course load. The an-

swer was no, that students should not be grading other students' work (even though this is a common practice for paid student assistants at other schools). He was not supportive regarding my vision change, and I truly believed that I could not ask for money from my employer to pay for accommodations I needed to do my job. Later, I asked if I could pay a student to read the textbook to me, since the print was too small. It was taking me many hours to read the book, as this was before I obtained a closed circuit television (CCTV). Having a student reader allowed me to rest my eyes and take notes and save some time in lecture preparation.

The inherent message I got from my supervisors at that school was downright wrong and illegal. I should have been more proactive in requesting accommodations, but I didn't know any better. About a year later, after I visited the STAR Center for a low vision exam (described in Chapter Six), I brought my accommodation request to the dean and bypassed my immediate supervisors. When the dean said yes to paying for a CCTV, I was so appreciative and excited that I almost bent down to kiss his shoe!

When I accepted a job offer at Allegheny College, I took a bold step and insisted that my accommodations be written into my job contract. I requested a CCTV for my office, costing about $3,000, separate from my laboratory research start-up funds. I was grateful to have a job during the 2009 recession, albeit a job with a greater workload than that at Lambuth. Employers are supposed to provide accommodations to employees as long as they are requested properly. The standard procedure is to obtain a doctor's letter explaining why they are needed in the workplace.

Requesting the CCTV was necessary because it is critical to my work. To read journal articles and textbooks, I routinely use a CCTV. To grade student assignments, I probably use the CCTV 25% of the total grading time. For many other activities, like operating a classroom computer, though, I use a hand-held magnifier.

At Columbus State Community College, the Department of Equity & Compliance was willing to work with me, and I met the coordinator of the office about six weeks after the semester started. I got a letter from my low vision doctor explaining the accommodations I needed. Sadly, because I was an adjunct faculty member, meaning a part-time instructor, it was decided that no resources would be purchased for my work. Since I wasn't given a computer that magnifies, I did my grading and lecture preparation at home rather than in the adjunct office, since at home I had the needed devices.

Computer Accommodations

When I started working at Allegheny College, the Microsoft operating system was standard issue, while the Apple operating system (Macintosh or Mac) was only by special request. I used Microsoft for many years, but as my disease progressed, I learned that Macs had higher ratings for accessibility. By 2016, I was convinced that a Mac would be more effective for my work, and so I asked for one. Thirteen months later, I was given a Mac, and it proved to be more productive. I really liked the accessibility features, such as holding down three keys (Alt, Apple symbol and +, or Option, Command and =) that enlarged the contents of the screen twofold. I discovered that this is a toggle feature, which means three keys (use - instead of +) reverse the enlargement back to normal size.

One of the frustrations I experienced with Microsoft was when I tried to open a Google Doc. Google Docs became a popular word processing program in academia in the early 2010s; it allows multiple users to edit a file simultaneously. However, this program was inaccessible on my Microsoft operating system for many years, and my supervisors used it routinely. When I tried to use a Google Doc, I got an error message that read, "The current window is too small to currently display this content." On multiple occasions, I was irrationally angry at this message and called Google's Technical Support to ask for assistance. The company was aware of the incompatibility issue but had no solution. They suggested I use an Apple computer system instead.

For a while, my response to this inaccessibility issue was denial. If someone sent me a file that I could not open, I told myself that it was not important and was something I could ignore. With all of the other challenges facing a faculty member, reading a few department files was low priority. Finally, when a Mac arrived in my office, it felt great to read and edit all the files that were shared with me.

Dealing with Administration
When I thought about my limitations, I felt inferior. This was not a conducive mindset for employment negotiations. I did not want to be "the squeaky wheel" when asking for assistance or accommodations.

At about the same time that my first contract renewal was being decided, the dean invited me to her office for a meeting "to discuss your vision." This was a foreboding request made by email, and my first thought was, "I'm going to be fired." I asked another administrator to attend the meeting as my advocate, to defend me if I was unable to defend myself.

The meeting went quite differently than I had anticipated. I was asked why students had never mentioned my vision on teaching evaluations. The short answer was that my vision was not an issue in the classroom. I do so many little things to compensate for what I cannot see. The students rarely notice, or, if they do, it is not detrimental to their learning. I was then asked to read a student evaluation comment. I explained that reading a student's handwriting of that size was impossible without magnification. So, the dean asked the director of Human Resources to read the comment aloud to us. It was an odd situation, having a near-stranger read a very personal comment aloud to three other people. At the conclusion of the meeting, the dean created an accommodation account for my future needs, and I was to make requests via the Human Resources director. Overall, it was a radical change from what I had expected. Ironically, the director was later diagnosed with age-related macular degeneration. It was nice to know we now had a true understanding of each other and what we were going through.

Asking for Other Accommodations

A few months after the first contract renewal, my vision worsened dramatically to an acuity of 20/150. At one of the lowest points in my life, at a party celebrating the beginning of the school year, I cried in front of the dean, sobbing about my vision and transportation challenges. I would not recommend doing this. However, the next month I made my first request to the director of Human Resources, for a magnifier to use at home. So much of my grading load required a magnifier. It seemed easier to grade at home. It was approved the next day by the dean. Maybe my emotional scene at the party was still in her memory.

Over the next few years, I asked for more accommodations at work, with three direct requests to the director of Human Resources. First, I needed a larger monitor, which allowed me to read more content on the screen without moving the cursor or my head so often. Thankfully, this request was granted within one year.

My other issues related to information shared at group meetings. With my research interests, I was expected to attend two or three department committee meetings every week. A common problem was when the leader of the group failed to send the information (for instance, a meeting agenda) in advance. The leader would either display the information from a projector at the meeting or provide a handout. In either case, I could not read the information and so felt excluded from the other members. Since Allegheny's default text size was 11 point, handouts were printed in this size, and I could not read them without a magnifier.

I asked if a handout in 14 point could be printed just for me, or if the meeting agenda could be sent via email with a few hours' notice. I thought these were reasonable requests, but I experienced pushback and resentment from some leaders. Routinely I would hear, "Oh, sorry, Christy, I forgot to make you an enlarged version." I tried to respond politely and did my best at the meeting, considering that I could not follow whatever was presented visually.

Since these problems continued through the next year, I asked the director of Human Resources to gently remind the leaders to please send agendas in advance in accessible formats. Overall, the situation improved, but it was only about 75% effective. I wondered, if a student with a vision problem like mine was in their class, would these leaders treat them in the same manner, apologizing for not meeting the accommodation? At least students had a forceful advocate who they could turn to for support: the director of Disability Services.

Co-worker Interactions

When my vision first began to worsen, while I worked at Lambuth University (January 2006), I decided not to tell all of my co-workers about it. Lambuth was a small community, and it seemed like I was living in a fishbowl with everyone watching me. My attitude was "need to know": "If they need to know, I will tell them." So, a few of my immediate co-workers were aware of my vision change, but the rest of the campus did not know. My personal information wasn't a secret, but it wasn't common knowledge, either.

At Allegheny College, I got a lesson in blindness awareness when my contract was first renewed, 18 months after I started teaching there. In the last paragraph of my self-evaluation, I wrote something like "Considering I cannot see student facial expressions, I think I am doing a good job." I learned later that my blindness was a major topic in the discussion of my job performance. The one quote that a tenured faculty member shared with me was, "How can she teach if she can't see the students' faces?" I believe this was a telling statement, indicating that at least several of the members of the Biology Department were biased against the disabled. In my opinion, seeing faces is a small part of the job of a teacher, and this factor can be overcome by a relationship that emphasizes verbal communication. However, I told myself that once my co-workers got to know me better, this bias would fade away.

In the next year, my visual acuity slipped to 20/110. I had connected with Vocational Rehabilitation (VR), part of the Bureau of Blindness and Visual Services (BBVS), Department of Labor & Industry, Commonwealth of Pennsylvania. Their office was focused on helping me maintain my job. I was assigned a fantastic caseworker named Rebecca, who proposed an Individualized Plan for Employment (IPE). This plan included three steps of counseling and guidance, a low vision evaluation and recommended aids, computer or assistive technology evaluation, and recommended equipment and training.

This plan provided me with a Macintosh laptop computer and magnification software for both my office and lab computers. My counselor also had a few ideas for improving my workplace environment. In terms of guidance, Rebecca and I agreed that she should speak on my behalf to my department colleagues, including the dean. She explained my vision disease, the challenges I was facing, and how they could be supportive.

I had hoped that my co-workers would feel more comfortable talking to me about my disease after that meeting. Sadly, this was only true for the 3 staff members and 2 of the 14 faculty members in the department. The majority of my colleagues, however, never mentioned my vision again. It became an uncomfortable topic. My plan had backfired.

While describing this situation to a colleague in the Philosophy Department, he noted that the topic of disability was "the elephant in the room," similar to the topic of race. It often results in people refusing to discuss it entirely in the future. In subsequent contract renewals, in the department's letters supporting my re-appointment, there was no mention of blindness or adjustments to work duties in regards to my changing vision.

A reader might ask, "Why did you want your co-workers to talk about your vision? Wouldn't you rather they focus on work instead of a personal problem?" The answer is that I wanted to feel accepted by my co-workers. Blindness is such an isolating disability. I felt that they were avoiding the topic because they were uncomfortable, which in turn made me uncomfortable with my own disease. I could not separate whether they disliked blind people or whether they just couldn't appreciate what I was facing.

One of my journal entries from July 2013 is pertinent:

I am currently debating whether to embrace the vision thing, making it more widely known, or to keep it to myself. There is such a stigma about vision loss, and literally everyone at the [VISIONS 2013] conference advised that revealing a vision problem to an employer is the kiss of death. I heard some employment horror stories. … On the other hand, the more we hide it, the longer it will take until it is accepted.

I also wanted to be understood, but now I realize that some people are not capable of understanding blindness. Some of them took a while to comprehend that I could not see them and that was the reason I was behaving differently than before. Kleege (1999, 35) observed, "…what you fear is not your inability to adapt to the loss of sight, it is the inability of people around you to see you the same way." Along with this perspective, Hull (1990, 58) pointed out, "Not to see is the same as not to be seen…. A blind person is invisible." The longer I worked at Allegheny College, the more I felt invisible to my co-workers. In hindsight, they didn't realize what they were doing was offensive.

Chapter Twelve
The Saga of Obtaining a Bioptic Driver's License

A friend asked me how long it had been since I stopped driving. "Five years," I replied. She said, "Oh, that's not such a long time." I looked at her and blurted, "Five years feels like an eternity!"

Can I Drive Again?
My bioptic driving journey began in the summer of 2015, during a visit with my optometrist, Dr. Dustin Mitchell, a then-recent graduate of The Ohio State University (OSU) College of Optometry. He referred me to a low vision doctor at his alma mater. My previous low vision exam had been several years earlier, with Dr. Andrew Prischak of The Erie Sight Center. It seemed like a good time for a low vision checkup and to learn about any devices that might help me.

The Low Vision Exam
When I met Dr. Roanne Flom at OSU in July 2015, she examined my eyes, noting that I had good peripheral vision and contrast sensitivity. Contrast sensitivity is a way to assess vision for drivers and pilots. The Air Force needs to verify that pilots can identify targets at a distance even under low contrast conditions (Ginsberg 1983, 15). It seems to be a better measure of vision than acuity. My acuity in both eyes was 20/120. In the previous

month with Dr. Mitchell, my acuity was recorded as 20/200. However, the discrepancy was only due to the charts used. Dr. Mitchell used a Snellen chart, while Dr. Flom used an ETDRS chart. Snellen eye charts have lines designated 100 and 200, whereas an ETDRS chart has lines at 120 and 150 as well, allowing for more precise measurement. Dr. Flom suggested that I use reading glasses to correct presbyopia when working on the computer. Presbyopia is farsightedness caused by natural aging of the lens. This can make it difficult to focus on small print, which happens for most people around age 40 and gets worse every ten years.

A quote from my journal entry that day reads, "Biggest news: she said I could train with bioptics to drive in Ohio!" Translation: Dr. Flom said that I was a good candidate for Ohio's Bioptic Driving Program. This was exciting and something to actually look forward to. I asked for more information, and she gave me a brochure about the Bureau of Services and Vision Impairment (BSVI). Still, I had doubts about whether I could complete the program. I really did not want to get my hopes up about driving in the future if I were likely to fail.

The factors that made me a good candidate for the Bioptic Driving Program included my good peripheral vision, my high contrast sensitivity and the fact that I had been a driver for over 20 years. Reading signs from a distance was my biggest challenge. With 20/120 acuity, I could usually read signs from the passenger seat just before I passed them. Dr. Flom said bioptic glasses could help me read signs from farther away, subsequently enabling me to drive again.

The first time I heard about bioptic driving was from an acquaintance with Stargardt disease living in California. She had been driving with bioptic glasses for years. At the time, I was living in the Commonwealth of Pennsylvania. Since Pennsylvania did not allow bioptics to be used for the driver vision test, I had not investigated that option.

What Is Bioptic Driving?

Bioptic driving allows some people with vision loss, such as albinism, macular degeneration, nystagmus and optic neuropathy, to drive with a special device. In Ohio, a policy change in 1990 allowed drivers to wear a miniaturized telescope to take the visual test. Prior to this date, drivers were allowed to take the visual test only with eyeglasses or contact lenses. The Bioptic Driving Program is certified by the Ohio Department of Highway Safety (Northern Ohio Bioptic Driving Program brochure 2018).

Known as a spectacle-mounted telescope, the bioptic is a telescopic lens attached to a carrier eyeglass frame. One example is shown in **Figure 11**. Most of the time, the user looks through the carrier lens for normal viewing, using the telescope for "quick spotting" when necessary (Chun, Cucuras and Jay 2016, 53). In the field of optics, the greater the optical power is, the smaller the field of view. This small field of view is appropriate for reading distant signs or identifying road obstacles. Bioptics are intended for viewing small objects in the distance, not a broad scene.

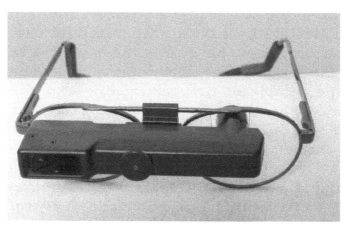

Figure 11: Keplerian-style telescopic glasses

There are seven steps for a candidate to earn his or her driver's license: a vision exam, bioptic telescope evaluation and fitting, evaluation of vision through bioptic telescope, training in bioptic use, written test of traffic laws and signs (that is, a driver permit), driver in-car training and an in-car test. The in-car training for adults who have driving experience is a minimum of 20 hours. For new drivers, it is a minimum of 40 hours for those over age 18 and 58 hours for those under age 18 (Northern Ohio Bioptic Driving Program brochure 2018).

There are more than 5,000 bioptic drivers in the United States. According to Chuck Huss, a Driver Rehabilitation Specialist in West Virginia in early 2022, bioptic telescopic glasses were allowed for driving in 48 states, the exceptions being Connecticut and Iowa; Utah added bioptic requirements recently. Although regulations vary by state, Ohio's rules appear similar to those of most other states that allow bioptic driving. Canada and the Netherlands also allow driving with bioptic glasses.

In the calendar year of 2018-2019 in Ohio, there were 31 potential drivers in the Bioptic Driving Program, the Records Department of the Ohio Bureau of Motor Vehicles informed me. There were 65 tests, with 43 passes and 22 failures. How do 31 clients result in 43 passed tests? A driver earns a daytime driving license by taking two tests. If the person fails the first test, he or she must wait a full year to re-take it. However, if the driver passes test #1, he or she completes driver training and takes test #2. So, a single client may have two passes in a year. If he or she fails test #2, the person can re-take it, but he or she does not need to wait a whole year for that. Lastly, a bioptic daytime driver may take the nighttime driving test after having the daytime license for one year. In other words, drivers need a full year of driving experience before attempting to drive at night. I think this is a reasonable policy.

Early Steps in Getting a License
I became an Ohio resident in early 2016 and called the Ohio BSVI for an intake appointment in Canton, Ohio. This site was closest to our home. Unfortunately, the first appointment was canceled due to employee illness, but I still paid $100 for a ride to Canton. The rescheduled intake was a fairly standard meeting with questions about me and my vision disease. The goal of the BSVI is to provide services to help residents gain employment or remain employed. The BSVI has changed its name since then; currently the agency is called Opportunities for Ohioans with Disabilities (OOD).

About six weeks after the intake appointment, I was approved by BSVI to meet with a low vision specialist in Akron. Apparently Dr. Flom's exam was insufficient because it occurred nine months earlier (ah, bureaucratic hurdles!). I met Dr. Cheryl Reed in May at the Judith A. Read Low Vision Services, which is part of United Disability Services (UDS). She performed a variety of tests, including contrast sensitivity, and determined that a Keplerian telescope would be the best option for me. The other type of bioptic telescope used is the Galilean style (www.ocutech.com).

In the next administrative step, I was approved by BSVI with a plan for the telescope, testing and driver training. The estimated price tag, paid by the State of Ohio, would be $2,500. I agreed to this plan, with the understanding that at any point in the process, I could be rejected from the program. If that were to happen, the program's policy was that a client must wait one year for a re-try. I also would have to return all of the items that the program ordered for me, like the bioptic glasses.

I was fitted for the Keplerian telescope and carrier frame during my second visit to Dr. Reed in June, and she placed the product order. The miniature telescope was positioned in the middle upper portion of the left lens of the carrier frame, where my best remaining vision was located. The glasses arrived in August, later than I had expected, after a few phone calls and a small donation to UDS. This was another lesson in patience, as there was no fast track to becoming a bioptic driver.

Training #1: Using Bioptic Glasses as a Passenger
There are two training stages: using the bioptic glasses as a passenger (#1) and actual in-car driving (#2). I met with the first instructor, Kim, who gave me written and oral instructions about what the bioptic vision test would entail. This seemed like a daunting task, and I wondered if I really could drive again. What if I failed?

The experience of wearing the bioptic glasses in the car differed from the brief time I was fitted with them in the doctor's office. First, they are heavy. My regular glasses (for myopia to provide distance vision) weigh 23 grams. My favorite pair of sunglasses weighs 37 grams, and the bioptic telescopic glasses weigh 74 grams, plus a 5-gram filter. So, there is a comfort issue, as the bioptic glasses frequently leave a mark on the bridge of my nose. It took some time to accustom myself to having this heavy frame on my face.

Second, I was supposed to use both eyes to see, but the telescope was positioned on the upper part of the left lens. I had to train myself to dip my head to look through the telescope with my left eye for one second and simultaneously not close my right eye. I am left-eye dominant, and my brain was accustomed to ignoring much of the information from my right eye. I reminded myself, "Keep your right eye open!" until it became a habit.

Initially, I didn't fully comprehend the instructions of the passenger training. If I could not drive with the glasses until I had a driver's license, what was I to do with them? Well, I was supposed to sit in the passenger seat and use the glasses **as if** I were driving. Instead of reading the signs at a distance of 20 feet, for instance, I could now read the signs from much farther away. A red stop sign was easy to recognize, but the glasses helped me to read the yellow signs with text or images, which might indicate a lane clo-sure or another impediment. Reading the green direction signs, especially the ones that indicate which lane to take for certain destinations, was much easier with the glasses.

Kim and I met for three sessions. The first was a run-through of what was expected in the vision test as a passenger. During the test, I was sup-posed to vocalize what I could see, including all of the relevant items that a driver encounters like road signs and traffic signals. I would indicate the color of the traffic signal by saying "Traffic sig-nal green." When brake lights of vehicles appeared, I said, "Brake lights on." At city intersections, I struggled with the white lane sign; this sign, for example, might have a left turn lane, middle lane going straight, and right turn lane. I needed prac-tice using verbal commands while wearing the glasses, and the many signs at city intersections were especially tough. I had not driven in big cit-ies by myself for many years. Also, after being only a passenger for five years and trusting the driv-er, I had begun to pay less attention to all those things. Finally, the instructions for test #1 includ-ed this statement: if the candidate failed any of the tests, he would need to wait a calendar year to resume training.

I failed the second session of the passenger test because I needed more practice with certain driving situations. One of the driving routes of the test was Market Street in Akron, which has about ten traffic signals over a stretch of two miles. I had developed a bad habit of dipping my head too often (about every 15 seconds), because I anticipated that it was time to use the glasses again. I had to learn that dipping and using the telescope was only needed when I saw an item in my peripheral vision that I wanted to see more clearly. My mistake was that I was trying to set a routine, but driving is often unpredictable. The driver needs to be aware at all times. No matter where I was driving, the telescope should not be used on a schedule!

I was quite nervous for the third session with Kim, but this time I passed! Although I was still not using the bioptics 100% appropriately, I was in the acceptable range.

Training #2: Driving the Car
After passing the first test (using the bioptic glasses as a passenger), the next step was getting a driver's learning permit. Kim gave me a copy of Ohio's Motor Vehicle Laws. A week later, I got a ride to the Bureau of Motor Vehicles (BMV) and passed the computerized test!

Next, I scheduled the long-awaited, in-car driver training. This was 20 hours in a car with Kathleen, the driver trainer at the Edwin Shaw Rehabilitation Center (now Cleveland Clinic Akron General Rehabilitation and Sports Therapy). Kathleen is an occupational therapist, and we drove a big, silver Buick sedan. We scheduled five, four-hour sessions, Monday through Friday in one week. Three of the days we met from 1 to 5 p.m., and 8 a.m. to noon on the remaining two. Fortunately, I was on sabbatical leave that semester, so the training did not conflict with my teaching schedule.

The first day of driver training went really well; we reviewed the three parts of the upcoming test. Part 1, passenger identification or spotting, is unique to bioptic training. For practice, we parked in a parking lot about 50 feet from a four-way intersection. Sitting in the passenger seat, I was asked to quickly describe what I saw using the telescope. For instance, I was asked to count how many cars were traveling east (to the right) through the intersection, the colors of the vehicles, and whether each vehicle was a car or truck. Part 2 was maneuverability and navigating an obstacle course, which included putting the car into forward and reverse around some orange cones. Part 3 was driving on roads. I wrote in my journal, "It felt good to finally be driving on the road." By the fourth day of in-car training, I was driving on highways!

After 20 hours of driver training, Kathleen thought I was ready for the test, and we scheduled it a few weeks later. Most drivers-in-training are allowed to drive with a registered driver sitting in the passenger seat. However, in the bioptic driver program, the rules are stated clearly: a bioptic driver-in-training is only allowed to drive with the trainer as passenger.

Driving Test

On the appointed morning, I met two highway patrol officers at the BMV. I adjusted the car mirrors and away we went. I passed the passenger identification test and the obstacle/mobility course. If a driver candidate fails either of these tests, the testing ends. Since I had anticipated failing one of them, I was not mentally prepared for the third test, the on-the-road driving. I was very excited to have reached the third test and was perhaps overly confident.

I failed the "driving-on-roads" portion. While much of the test was a breeze, there were three problem areas. In a neighborhood with stop signs on every block, I did not spend enough time bringing the car to a complete stop. This was a bad habit I had developed in my younger years. I drove above the speed limit past a cemetery with a 30 mph zone. Finally, when we got on the highway, I drove too fast again.

Although I failed my first driving test, overall I felt pretty good about myself. We scheduled a second test two weeks later. It would have been nice to go the next day, but the wait time was not a big deal. I had already waited five years for this driving opportunity. I passed all three tests on my second attempt! **Figure 12** shows a photograph of me in my vehicle with my bioptic glasses and a black filter.

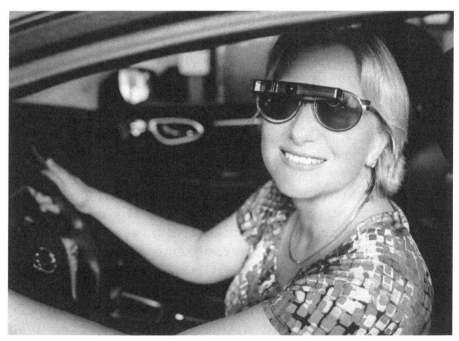

Figure 12: Photo of me in my car

Bioptic Driving Program Summary
All in all, there were many hurdles and delays in getting a bioptic driver's license. The program was effective, but it took longer than I had hoped. I am glad the program was rigorous, testing visual, cognitive and motor skills. It gave me the time to boost my confidence and pass each test.

Observations about Driving with Bioptic Telescopic Glasses

Visibility is important when you are a bioptic driver. Unfortunately, when the weather is gray and cloudy with rain or snow, bioptic glasses do not help much. These are considered poor driving conditions, and it is important to decide whether driving is really necessary. At one point I thought my vision was changing. Then I realized that the car windshield was dirty. What a relief when I cleaned the windshield and could see clearly! On sunny days, I use a black filter, shaped like the two lenses, with a hole punched into it to fit over the telescope. This helps to minimize the glare.

The glasses require little maintenance. When I am not wearing them, I put the bioptic glasses in a sturdy container provided by the manufacturer. Cleaning them is important.

Show and Tell

I used my bioptic glasses in a show-and-tell format for some of my classes. Students tried them on and looked at a distant point. Not everyone "got it," but many did. It was an important experience for the students to understand how a visually-impaired person can be assisted in gaining his or her independence.

Appearances

I was very self-conscious of how the bioptic glasses looked on my face. I thought I looked like a weirdo, but it was a trade-off between appearance and function. Did it matter what I looked like if I could see what everyone else can see?

I became less self-conscious about six months after earning my license. They became a tool that I was proud of and not something to hide. I even wore them in a work meeting with colleagues!

Cost Comparison

Transportation cost is something that most people do not consider—at least until their vehicle is getting major repairs. It was a major expense for me. In 2014, when I was dating long-distance, I spent between $100 and $200 per weekend for a ride to and from Ohio, a one-way trip of 140 miles. If I visited my boyfriend three times in a month, the total could be $600. Once I got my bioptic driver's license, those costs went down. In July 2017, I drove three times from my house to my workplace in Meadville (and back). Paying for a car loan, auto insurance and fuel totaled about $400 per month. However, because I had the vehicle at my disposal for the rest of the month, it was a huge lifestyle change in terms of convenience. The independence of being able to drive and run errands during daytime hours was liberating!

Driving Highlights and Lowlights

A few months after earning my driver's license, I drove about 500 miles in one day, from Ohio to Nashville, Tennessee, by myself. It took seven and a half hours, and I took regular breaks at rest areas and followed the posted speed limits. I was lucky to avoid driving west directly into the glare of the setting sun.

Global Positioning Systems (GPS) are effective driving aids, especially for visiting a new site. Chun, Cucuras and Jay (2016, 56) say they can be used "to prepare for lane changes and turns." Although I don't trust it 100% of the time, it can really help in navigation while I focus on the road.

During the first eight months after I earned my license, I would wake up and wonder if today would be my last day of driving. If that was just fear, it did not last long, and one day I realized that I began taking my driving privileges for granted again. In my second year of driving, I got two speeding tickets, obtained from posted cameras above Interstate 80. I haven't actually been pulled over by a police officer, so I'm not sure how that sort of interaction might go.

Non-Driving Purposes

I have worn the bioptic glasses in a few non-driving situations. I wear them during my church's worship services, which allows me to read the projected song lyrics. This makes me feel like a part of the group. I am still self-conscious about my appearance, so I sit toward the back of the room, minimizing how many people see me in my funny glasses.

I also wore them to a science conference in order to read presentation slides. It was a moment that changed how I approached those kinds of gatherings. I was able to fully appreciate the presentation, as I could when my acuity was 20/30. I was less self-conscious in a room of 200 strangers, as scientists generally do not care about appearance.

A low vision doctor told me that one patient uses the bioptic glasses to watch television. Perhaps I am accustomed to watching TV without glasses, and sharp focus is not important to me. However, I should try wearing them to watch a foreign film at a movie theater. Maybe I will be able to read the subtitles!

Pennsylvania

After earning my Ohio driver's license in 2017, I considered moving closer to my workplace in Pennsylvania. I called Pennsylvania's Department of Motor Vehicles (DMV) and asked about transferring my bioptic driver's license. I was told unequivocally that my Ohio driver's license would be revoked if I became a Pennsylvania resident. This important milestone was not something that I wanted to lose.

Chun, Cucuras and Jay (2016, 56) noted that Pennsylvania is in the category of states that allow bioptic glasses to be used to drive as a visual aid but that require the vision standards be passed without them. This seems strange to me. If you expect a person to drive with contact lenses, then the person takes the vision test with the contact lenses. Other states that share this view include Florida, Hawaii, Missouri, New Mexico and Wisconsin. At that time thirty-seven states allowed bioptics in vision tests for driving.

In November of 2020, the Pennsylvania governor signed HB2296 into law, aiming for implementation in Fall 2021. Chuck Huss informed me about this law. This legislation finally allows some low vision patients to drive with bioptic glasses. It requires 10 hours of passenger-in-car training and 20 hours of behind-the-wheel training, with appropriate trainers, plus 45 hours of additional training. There are more restrictions than what Ohio requires of its bioptic drivers, like a radius of driving from home and no interstate driving. My personal opinion is that this is a good first step, but I would hate those particular restrictions. I love driving on interstate highways and do it very well!

Final Thought
Maybe ten years from now (or sooner), self-driving cars will be safe and commonplace. Maybe the cost will be reasonable for visually-impaired individuals to purchase them. However, until that day comes, I am appreciative of the bioptic training program and the freedom that I have gained.

Chapter Thirteen
Disability and the Blind Community

Early Interactions with Blind People

Prior to my macular degeneration diagnosis, I had little personal experience with anyone who was blind. None of my older family members during my childhood had serious eye problems. The only blind teacher I encountered in over 18 years of education was a professor of U.S. History. Around campus, there was a rumor that he had bad vision and students were advised to write large and neatly in their blue books on exams. Perhaps he had macular degeneration.

As it was for me in my younger years, many people have never interacted with a blind person, and "they have little idea of what to do or how to relate" (Hull 1990, 110). The first time I was in a social situation with a blind person, I struggled to find something to talk about and avoided some topics. It did not occur to me, then, that the person was like me, having a variety of interests such as music, sports and current events.

After meeting other blind people, I became more comfortable talking with them. I reminded myself that they are people who want to be treated with respect, just like me. Although our experiences with vision loss may differ, there are plenty of commonalities and things to talk about.

Blind people sometimes complain about comments made by sighted people, I used to hear someone say, "I can't imagine what you are going through!" Sometimes I want to reply that their imaginations are lacking. All you would need to do is close your eyes for a few hours to feel what it is like to be blind. Sighted people may feel pity, charity, admiration or scorn for the blind (Kleege 1999, 3). Rothschild is amused by comments about her courage for being blind (2002, 52).

In another observation, "Some [people] even romanticize it, marveling at how 'perceptive' I must be or how acute my other senses are" (Rothschild 2002, 141). Many blind people are annoyed by this view, and, like me, have learned to tolerate it. Let me emphasize that my sense of hearing has not improved since my vision began to fail. I still cannot distinguish voices very well. Instead, I just utilize my hearing more than I used to because my vision is not dependable. Finally, I am amused when people comment about how much courage a blind person exhibits. What makes me courageous has nothing to do with my vision or whether I get out of bed to face the world every day. Rather, this is what people say politely when they cannot think of anything else to say that is nice or genuine.

How to Give Directions
When giving directions to a blind person, it is okay to use "left" and "right" to describe objects ahead. A common analogy for describing food on a plate is to use a clock. For example, "The carrots are at three o'clock." (Of course, with digital display technology replacing old-fashioned clocks, fewer people are able to read the hands of a clock, and this method may fail in the future.) If one is walking with a blind person, the sighted individual should offer an elbow and allow the blind person to hold onto it.

The Word "Blind"

The words "blind" and "blindness" refer to lack of sight, but they are somewhat unclear. Total blindness means not being able to perceive light, which is what ophthalmologists call no light perception (NLP). Sight represents a spectrum from fully sighted to totally blind, and it is not an all-ornothing situation. About 15% of blind individuals are completely blind, and the rest of us have some level of usable vision. A better descriptor for those in the middle of the spectrum is "partially sighted." "Blind" might be an insufficient term, but it is a simple word that suggests something is wrong with the eyes or the part of the brain receiving information from the eyes.

I am partially sighted and not blind and often use the phrase "visually-impaired." Those two words are still a little bulky and not clear to everyone, so sometimes it is just easier to say that I am blind. If I am speaking with a stranger, he or she may give me a quizzical look because my appearance does not match the person's expectation. On several occasions others have asked the question, "How can you be blind if you are making eye contact?" I am pretty good at making eye contact, or at least appearing to. I had years of practice before I lost my central vision.

One of the current debates in the blind community is whether to use the term "visually-impaired" or "visually-challenged," suggesting that the latter is a more positive expression. As stated earlier, I lean toward using "visually-impaired," but perhaps I will switch to "visually-challenged" in the future. Whether I use "partially sighted," "visually-impaired" or "visually-challenged," all of these terms still require further clarification. What objects can I see and what can't I see? One of my friends teases me that I should wear a yellow "I have low vision" button. But "low vision" is another term that many sighted individuals are not familiar with. Maybe we just need a way to educate everyone on these definitions.

There is a debate in the disability field about words and word order when referring to a person. Should the disability be mentioned first or second? For instance, am I a visually-impaired person or a person with a visual impairment? The experts refer to this as person-first or disability-first language. When I'm in a hurry, I use the former term because it's shorter. Since I like to remind myself that I am a person first and my disability is a secondary trait, I like the latter term, too. Another troublesome phrase is "people with disabilities." This is too general and runs into similar problems as using the phrase "people of color." Grouping a deaf person and a person who uses a wheelchair with blind people is sometimes useful, but there are many differences among the groups.

Legal Blindness

The criteria for legal blindness is either having best corrected visual acuity (BCV) of 20/200 (or worse) or having a visual field of 10 degrees or less. The latter condition is referred to as peripheral loss. This is a common symptom of patients with retinitis pigmentosa. For the first category, a policy change occurred in 2007. Using an ETDRS chart, a patient with visual acuity worse than 20/100 meets the criterion of legal blindness. According to Wikipedia, about 3.4 million Americans have low vision, and the majority of those individuals are legally blind.

Since 2011, I had been convinced that I was not legally blind because my acuity was around 20/150. Maybe that doctor should have been explicit, saying, "You are legally blind now." Ironically, I learned about the legal blindness policy change in the year 2020 while writing this book.

Blindness Strikes All Walks of Life

"We all come to blindness at different times in our lives and from different backgrounds and perspectives" (Frederick 2016). Blindness is an equal opportunity disability. It happens to the rich and the poor of all races. However, if I were blind and wealthy, my life would be substantially different than that of a poor blind person.

Belonging to a Community

At age 30, I did not feel like I belonged to the age-related macular degeneration (AMD) community. Even at age 40, I thought I had little in common with them. It seemed that AMD patients were dealing with end-of-life issues, whereas I was trying to maintain a job. When I interacted with clients of the Keystone Blind Association, I learned that we do have some things in common. We share the issues of not seeing well and encountering sighted people who do not understand us. Instead of being "like everyone else," I had to accept my different capabilities. This change in identity was a switch from being an average person to being a minority, someone outside the normal group.

Another Disabled Group

The deaf community is interesting in comparison to the blind community. As I learned from Leah Cohen's book, *Train Go Sorry* (1994), deaf people are a tightly knit group of about 2 million Americans, having their own social clubs and athletic leagues. Most deaf children are born to hearing parents, so they learn deaf culture in deaf schools. In the United States, they have their own language, American Sign Language (ASL). Until the 1960s, ASL was not considered a legitimate language, mainly because using hand signals was thought to be primitive. For decades, deaf people were taught an oralist education where they learned to speak and read lips, which was believed by many advocates to help deaf individuals succeed in society.

There have been many strides in educational and public policy related to the deaf community, particularly from 1970 to 1995. Many in the deaf community feel threatened by cochlear implants and a loss of deaf schools. The numbers of both deaf and blind children are decreasing due to a reduction in meningitis (the most common cause of deafness in children) and the adoption of cochlear implants.

Disability in General

When transitioning to the broader term of "disability" instead of "blindness," there are similar problems with definitions. The word "disability" suggests lack of ability, a status that is less than the normal experience. Like the word "blind," the words "disability" and "disabled" cannot specify to what extent that ability is altered or impaired. The term "differently abled" is not much better, in my opinion.

My introduction to the disabled world was through my employer. When my institution hired a new chief diversity officer in 2014, I scheduled a private meeting with her. At this point, I had lost enough vision to display 20/110 acuity, but I was still confused as to my status in terms of disability, as I was still following the old definition of 20/200 is legally blind. After explaining the progression of my vision disease in regards to my employment, I asked her, "Am I disabled?" Perhaps it is odd that I would ask a stranger about my status. Put simply, no one—not my eye doctor or my Vocational Rehabilitation counselor—had ever used the word "disabled" to describe me.

In 2014, I thought that "disabled" was equivalent to "legal blindness." If this were true, then I was not disabled. By the end of our conversation, however, we agreed that the term did, in fact, apply to me. I then began a new path: life with the label of disabled.

New Identity

"Disabled" is indeed a label. I'm not sure which term is less stigmatizing, "blind" or "disabled." They are both terms that the majority of people would prefer to avoid in their lifetimes. However, for the rest of my life I will be considered a disabled person by the government. When applying for jobs, I check the disabled box on the Equal Employment Opportunity (EEO) form. In addition, I became acutely aware of the stigma of disabled people in the workplace.

To satisfy my intellectual curiosity, I searched for reading material in the area of disability studies. I had never given much thought to how disabled people managed in our society. I had no idea what blind people did to accomplish tasks that regularly involved vision. One example of a visual task, to my understanding, was counting paper money. I learned that when a money bill is given to a blind person, he folds it in a certain way to indicate a $1, $5, $10 or $20 bill. Folding one corner makes a tactile difference between bills, which a blind person can distinguish.

Blind Assistance Agencies

If someone is blind from birth, there are a host of agencies that assist the child's parents. Those agencies have a variety of names, so it would be wise to consult a local ophthalmologist or Office of Human Services (or the state equivalent). A typical education of a blind child involves learning Braille at a school for the blind.

For an adult who becomes blind or visually-impaired, there are other agencies that assist. I believe that my family, friends and colleagues assumed that there was some government agency that "handles" people who develop blindness. These agencies do not contact the patient or seek out their clients, as there is no mechanism in place for them to get that kind of personal information. Instead, the patient must be the one to contact the agency for assistance. This was not initially clear to me. How does one find the right agency to ask for help? Sadly, word of mouth is the key component in finding community resources for the blind, and I did not know other blind people in my community.

Invisible Disability (ID)

One of my colleagues referred to me as having an invisible disability. I disliked the term, but it is true. My disability is invisible to most people. Because I appear to make eye contact when speaking to people, people do not realize that I cannot see them clearly. This is a blessing and a curse, a boon and a challenge. Having a disability that is not obvious to others allows me to hide in plain sight, if you pardon the pun. I can pretend to be able, to be like everyone else, until a visual test is applied. In fact, I regularly need to remind people that I cannot see something that everyone else in the room can see.

"Invisible disability" is a much broader and more inclusive term than I realized. According to the Invisible Disabilities Association (IDA, www.invisibledisabilities.org), an invisible disability is a limitation on activity and participation. Conditions such as psychiatric disorders, learning disabilities, HIV/AIDS, diabetes, heart disease and epilepsy are invisible disabilities. Of the total number of disabled people, about half have invisible disabilities. According to 2014 U.S. Census data on Americans with disabilities, 12.3 million individuals had difficulty seeing and 17 million individuals had difficulty hearing. From the 45 million adults over the age

of 65, 9.4% had difficulty seeing and 20% had difficulty hearing, with 39% having difficulty climbing
stairs and 2.3% using a wheelchair.

Returning to the chief diversity officer at my institution once more, she made an interesting sug-
gestion. I was seeking a support group, people at
my workplace who were disabled or at least different from the regular employees. First, she suggested I contact a counselor to discuss my feelings,
which I had done for several years when my vision
loss progressed. Then she encouraged me to attend meetings of the Lesbian-Gay-Bisexual-Transgender-Queer (LGBTQ) faculty group. I was initially
confused by this invitation. The LGBTQ group is a
minority group with some similarities to the disabled. Their differences of sexual orientation and
identity may be invisible to the majority group,
just as my blindness is invisible to my co-workers. What makes them different is their sexuality,
which is generally not obvious in the workplace.
My visual impairment is likewise hard to detect.

In both cases, there is a decision that individuals of these groups must make, whether "to come
out or to pass" in a social situation. Should I tell
a person who I just met that I have a visual impairment? Does the person need to know this personal information? Sometimes it is fine to share
it while other times I choose not to share it. My
problem with the comparison of disability to the
LGBTQ community is that being part of the LGBTQ
community is not a limitation in ability, such as
blindness or deafness. It was not the minority status that I struggled with in the workplace but the
limitations of my abilities.

The Privilege of Not Being Disabled
One semester I taught undergraduate students
about social justice. Together we learned about the
theoretical aspects regarding the differences that

disabled persons experience in society. In one of our readings, author Allan Johnson (2006) listed items attributed to privileged persons relative to persons with a disability: "Nondisabled people can assume that they will fit in at work and in other settings without having to worry about being evaluated and judged according to preconceived notions and stereotypes about people with disabilities" (30). In another example, he says, "Nondisabled people can go to polling places on election day knowing they will have access to voting machines that allow them to exercise their rights as citizens in privacy without the assistance of others" (Johnson 2006, 31). At the conclusion of this brief section in class, I was able to speak from my own experience of blindness, and students made the appropriate connections to their schoolwork.

How People Treat the Disabled

Beyond blindness, I think many people avoid people with a disability because they are unsure of how to act. John Hull (1990, 107), who lost all of his vision as a young adult, said, "Being disabled leads to people treating you like a child." This statement probably applies to some disabled people, but not all of us. Since I am partially sighted and can pretend to make eye contact, I am fortunately not treated as a child, at least not often. Other disabled people may feel invisible to the world or be considered asexual or unintelligent (Johnson 2006, 30).

When passing a person in a wheelchair, one of the issues I struggle with is whether to offer assistance at a doorway. Is it rude to offer help? This is an assumption that abled persons make, and, in this case, I am abled in regard to my walking ability. If the recipient could consider my offer rude, I try to make it in a way that is helpful and not condescending.

Entitled Disabled Persons

Over the years, I have encountered very few disabled people like myself in the workplace. I have met a few disabled students, two of whom are worth describing. The first carried an attitude of "other people should do things for me because I am incapable." Instead of finding ways to complete a task, this student expected others to do it for her. I think this is a variation of the millennial notion that "others should appreciate that I am gracing them with my presence." Unfortunately, as with so many groups, a few bad apples can ruin it for the rest of us. The other student had more than a few disabilities, yet she managed to solve problems independently. Excellent at solving problems is what I aspire to be.

Final Perspective

I am reminded of a TED talk by Chris Downey (2013), a man who suddenly became blind after brain surgery. He shared a statement from those in the disability field: "There are two types of people, those with a disability and those that have not found theirs yet." If we all will experience a disability in our lifetimes, then developing accessible technology and designing living and working environments should be priorities in human health.

Afterword

This work has been a journey of self-exploration. The initial concept came to me in July 2011, while riding an Amtrak train from Manhattan to Harrisburg. The outline I wrote that day has been reorganized many times, and the actual writing came in irregular spurts. One sunny day in May 2014, much of Chapter One, the story of my diagnosis, poured from my fingers onto the laptop keyboard. During semesters, I collected information and jotted down thoughts, which later became bits and pieces of chapters. It has taken me years to really commit to writing my story. There were many other projects and collaborations that I was asked to work on, so I put my own personal project to the side. By 2019, I decided that it was time to devote much more of my time to this work.

The work I wanted to write would be targeted toward non-scientists, those of the general public who were concerned with macular degeneration. The only currently available reading materials I found on this topic consisted of brochures found in medical offices and short descriptions on websites. Little else was geared toward patients or their friends and family. Since my intended scope was longer than a brochure, writing a book was the obvious choice.

When I told my academic friends of my early ideas of writing a book about my experience with vision loss, one of the common responses I received was, "Write a book? Why would you, a scientist, want to write a book?" In the natural sciences, the main form of publication is a primary article in a scientific journal, reporting an original experiment. I have written and published numerous primary articles based on original laboratory work, known as wet lab experiments. However, the book I was proposing was not based on lab experiments but rather my real-life story.

Few academic scientists pursue this direction because it is subjective instead of objective. I wanted to explain macular degeneration from both the scientific and patient perspectives. My goal also was to include some tidbits of optometry and ophthalmology and connect them with how patients actually experience macular degeneration. I knew that explaining this practical aspect would be useful, as well.

Many of the chapters of this book were heavily revised in the winter and spring of 2020. In April, I realized that what I had been drafting was actually two books. The other book is geared toward the science-health crowd; its working title so far is *The Real Story Behind Macular Degeneration*. It contains information about quality of life, supplements, vitamin A, how the eye works, aging diseases of the eye and DNA and genetic testing. It places more emphasis on future treatments of these diseases.

Finally, in the fall of 2020, I had two experiences that gave me the impetus to finish writing. I revisited Destin, Florida's white sandy beach with my husband, and this time there was no crying. Then, at the end of an exam with a retina specialist, the doctor said, "You probably know more about Stargardt disease than I do." I was disappointed, as I had hoped to learn more about my disease. However, this statement spurred me to finish the book and solicit a publisher.

I was successful.

Retinal Research Haiku
By Donald Gallick

Retinas will need light.
Retinal cells die, then darkness.
Cell death must end; how?

Glossary and Abbreviations

This section is needed because, as a biomedical scientist, I use abbreviations regularly, and the reader needs a reference point. I got this idea from a book about Lewy Body Dementia.

Glossary

Eye Anatomy

choroid: Blood supply to the retina

cone: A photoreceptor cell that detects a certain range of colored light

fovea: Central region of the macula with many cones

macula: Central region of the retina

optic nerve: Bundles of axons that carry visual information to the brain

photoreceptor: Cell that can absorb light rays and generate a cellular response

retina: Region of neurons at the back of the eye responsible for transforming light into a chemical signal and transmission of visual information

retinal pigment epithelium: A layer of cells between the choroid and neural retina

rod: An abundant photoreceptor

vitreous humor: Gel-like fluid between the lens and retina

Other Terms

carotenoids: Class of molecules of which several are used in the eye to absorb light

central vision loss: General term for conditions that result in damage to the macula while peripheral vision remains intact

contrast sensitivity: A measure of vision beyond acuity

dilation: Widening, in reference to the pupil

drusen: Yellowish deposits under the retina made of cellular debris

glaucoma: Vision disease in which aqueous humor accumulates and impairs ganglion cell signaling through the optic nerve

inflammation: General process by which body responds to damage or invasion

legal blindness: A term describing either worse than 20/100 acuity or having a 10-degree visual field in the better eye

lipofuscin: Molecule within retinal drusen thought to be responsible for damaged photoreceptors

lutein: Carotenoid found in the macula, included in AREDS2 formula

macular degeneration: A disease in which cells of the macula die

macular dystrophy: A collection of genetic diseases resulting in damage to the macula

myopia: Eye condition in which the focusing power of the cornea or lens is too strong

ophthalmoscope: An instrument used to view the retina and other parts of the eye

peripheral vision: Part of visual field that is not central

photophobia: Extreme sensitivity to light

presbyopia: Vision disease affecting people over age 40, reducing near vision

rhodopsin: Most abundant protein in the rod, capable of absorbing light

vitamin A: Molecule that generates the light-absorbing portion of rhodopsin

vitrectomy: A surgery in which the vitreous humor is removed and replaced with fluid and/or gas bubble

wet AMD: The more severe type of age-related macular degeneration that often results in large-scale vision loss

zeaxanthin: Carotenoid found in the macula, included in AREDS2 formula

Abbreviations

A2E: A molecule that can accumulate in retinal cells

ABCA4: ATP-binding cassette type 4, the current name of the gene responsible for Stargardt disease

ABCR: ATP-binding cassette transporter in retina, the original name for the gene that is mutated in Stargardt disease; the current abbreviation is ABCA4

AFB: American Federation of the Blind

AIDS: Acquired immunodeficiency syndrome

AMD: Age-related macular degeneration

AREDS2: Age-related eye disease study

ARMD: Less common abbreviation for age-related macular degeneration

ASL: American Sign Language

ATP: Adenosine triphosphate, a molecule used for cellular energy, allowing cells to do things like moving molecules across the cell membrane

BBVS: Bureau of Blindness and Visual Services (PA)

BCV: Best corrected visual acuity

BMV: Bureau of Motor Vehicles (OH)

BSVI: Bureau of Services and Vision Impairment (OH)

CATA: Crawford Area Transit Authority in Meadville, PA

CBS: Charles Bonnet syndrome

CCT: Cone contrast test

CCTV: Closed-circuit television

CFH: Complement factor H, a gene responsible for some cases of AMD

CNV: Choroidal neovascularization, known as wet AMD

CS: Contrast sensitivity

EEO: Equal Employment Opportunity, a government office

ELOVL4: Elongation of very long chain fatty acids type 4, a gene responsible for a subset of Stargardt disease

ETDRS: Early Treatment Diabetic Retinopathy Study

FA: Fluorescein angiogram, a test using a dye to identify retinal blood vessels

FFB: The Foundation Fighting Blindness, a non-profit organization raising funds for research on inherited retinal diseases

GA: Geographic atrophy, or advanced dry AMD

GPS: Global Positioning Systems

HIV: Human immunodeficiency virus

ID: Invisible disability

IDA: Invisible Disabilities Association

IOP: Intraocular pressure

IPE: Individualized Plan for Employment

IRDs: Inherited Retinal Diseases

KBA: Keystone Blind Association, a non-profit organization of Pennsylvania that provides several services

L-DOPA: A precursor molecule to the neurotransmitter dopamine

LGBTQ: Lesbian-Gay-Bisexual-Transgender-Queer group

MTA: Metro Transit Authority in New York City

NLP: No light perception

OCT: Optical coherence tomography, a test to display a cross-section of the retina, helpful in evaluating macular changes

OD: Oculis dexterous

O & M: Orientation and mobility, a training program especially for people with peripheral vision loss

OOD: Opportunities for Ohioans with Disabilities (OH)

OS: Oculis sinister

OSU: The Ohio State University

PED: Pigment epithelial detachment, a form of wet AMD

RPE: Retinal pigment epithelium

STGD: Stargardt disease, a form of macular degeneration that strikes patients before age 50

UDS: United Disability Services (OH)

VEGF: Vascular endothelial growth factor

VR: Vocational Rehabilitation (PA)

Acknowledgments

Inspiration from Other Writers
Initially, I was opposed to writing a memoir. I believed that memoirs are what celebrities write after a long career, and, surely, I am not a celebrity. Memoirs also can be written after a significant event, and, again, I did not think my life had a significant event that was worthy of writing a book. However, while preparing this book, I read a few memoirs. Those by Michael J. Fox, Jill Bolte Taylor and Marla Runyan resonated with me. Fox (2002) discussed his Parkinson's disease diagnosis and how it impacted his life. Bolte Taylor (2006) was a neuroanatomist by training and described her experience of a stroke from both the patient and scientist perspectives. Runyan (2001), a Stargardt patient, told her story of winning an Olympic medal in track and field.

I enjoyed reading Michael Deaver's memoir, *A Different Drummer* (2001), about Ronald Reagan. Deaver did not follow chronology. He discussed five years of service with the president before explaining the 1981 assassination attempt, which of course happened in the first year of Reagan's presidency. This order did not harm the story. Thus, I realized that chronological order was not absolutely necessary for my work. Instead, the order I chose emphasized my points.

Help from Many People
I have many people to thank for many types of contributions.

Thank you to Rosemary and Jim Worley, who supported me emotionally and spiritually during graduate school. Thank you to my mentors Owen McGuinness and David Wasserman at Vanderbilt University and John Nickerson from Emory Eye Center. John pointed me in the direction of studying why photoreceptors degenerate in a mouse model. One of my students, Jay Bruce, presented a talk entitled "Live and Let Die: The James Bond Approach to Photoreceptors."

Over the years, I have learned clinical information from retina specialists (MDs) J. Donald Gass, Anita Agarwal, Herbert Schubert and Alex Iannaconne. I have learned much from optometrists (ODs) Andrew Prischak, Sue Godzik, Christopher Adsit, Dustin Mitchell, Roanne Flom and Cheryl Reed.

Thank you to family and friends who offered support: Corinne Stockman, Nancy Fierer, Art Worley, Barbara Penn, Dana McCall, Carolynn and Robert Remington, Elizabeth Trabue, Karen Ko, Cindy Price, Debbie Stanger, Sara Lute and Janice Gorman.

Thank you to Veronica Schuver for connecting me with the talented Bryce Olson and suggesting that he might be interested in illustrating for this book. Thank you to Alexis Crump for her o-mamori, a Japanese eye health charm. Thank you to Paula Brownyard for referring me to the STAR Center and encouraging me to seek help for my vision. Thank you to former colleagues from Allegheny College who had positive impacts on my life with a vision impairment: Shafiq Rahman, Eleanor Weisman, Dave Roncolato, and Beth Watkins.

Thank you to Connie Ross for introducing me to her next-door neighbors Charlie and Mitzi Cummings. Thank you to Tammy Rozak and Megan Busson for opening the Doylestown Coffee House where I revised the manuscript. Thank you to Barbara Cordle, who introduced me to the term "godincidents." Thank you to Jen Harris for organizing a book signing.

Thank you to Marsha Blessing of Orison Publishers and editor Jeanette Sprecher.

The Writing Process

There were many people who offered feedback on the writing.

This book took shape from early discussions with Peggy Mitchell, Don Skinner and Allison Connell-Pinskey. Allison offered critical feedback about my audience while. Don helped me realize that I must be malleable, willing to give up some items as well as to fight for the right word.

Thank you to Kathleen Haskett for suggesting that my work be separated into a memoir and then a book geared toward health and science. As complicated as this idea seemed, it was the right way to approach what I wanted to do. Thank you to Dennis Murphy and Bob George of Keystone Blind Association for pointing out the need to separate dense scientific material into smaller, more manageable pieces.

Thank you to Chuck Huss and Kathleen Miller for feedback about bioptic driving programs in Ohio and other states.

Many others read certain chapters and provided proofreading assistance and feedback.

Thanks to the following family members: Carol Donmoyer, Carl and Susanne Donmoyer, Chuck Worley, Tara Sullivan and Rachel Stockman.

Thank you to the following friends: Stacey Dutt, Kim Barnett, Pastor Angela Lewis, Jeannette and Jim Hafey, Debbie and Keith Mink, Vicki Pope and Lin Sutley.

Thank you to some of my former Allegheny College students: Molly Proud (now OD), Alexis Crump, Stasia Georgiades, Veronica Schuver (now OD), Samuel Thomas, Terra Schall, Justine Kelly-Demello,

Cassie Dodson, Urszula Osczcapinska, Jorge Olan, Sami Landgraf, Julie Cepec, Spencer Braunstein, Patty Gaxiola, Jasmine Ramirez-Soto and Ryan Martinez. Thank you to Justin King (now MD), my favorite advisee from Lambuth University. Thank you to Eli Kirkendall from Columbus State Community College.

The more I learn about the eye and eye diseases, the more curious I become. I cannot recall where I learned every tidbit, but it has been a journey of information over two decades, and many eye health professionals have shared their knowledge with me along the way. Because I am not a clinician, I was anxious about sections that related to clinical practice. Several optometrists proofread various sections, including Molly Proud, Andrew Prischak, Sue Godzik, Dustin Mitchell, Veronica Schuver and John O'Donnell, Jr.

Thank you to Bryce Olson, who contributed four illustrations. I met Bryce in a class at Allegheny College, and his artistic talent was legendary.

Big thanks go to the people who proofread large portions of my writing: Peggy Mitchell, Charlie Cummings, Adrienne Perl, Polly Worley, Mary Jo Sullivan-Worley and Stasia Georgiades. Peggy Mitchel was my go-to person for all sorts of questions about blindness and disability. Charlie Cummings told me about the Akron Blind Center. He offered monthly feedback throughout the winter of 2019-2020, and he graciously loaned me Leah Cohen's book about the deaf community.

Thanks to My Husband
Finally, thank you to my husband Donald Gallick, who supported us when I chose to write full-time. He wrote the Photoreceptor Haiku used to introduce my research to undergraduates. He is the most wonderful combination of intelligence, caring, strength and wit. I am a lucky woman because

he makes me laugh every day. It is so much easier to get through life's rough patches when a laugh is around the corner.

Reference List

Chapter One: My Diagnosis Story

Pearce, J. 2005. "J. Donald M. Gass, 76, a Leading Ophthalmologist, Dies." *New York Times*, March 4.

Saunders, A. 1957. *Reader's Digest*. January.

Turbert, D. 2020. "What Is Histoplasmosis?" American Academy of Opthalmology. September 29. https://www.aao.org/eye-health/diseases/what-is-histoplasmosis.

Chapter Two: Coping with a Macular Degeneration Diagnosis

Bozarth, A. R. 1982. *Life Is Goodbye Life Is Hello: Grieving Well Through All Kinds of Loss*. Center City, Minnesota: Hazelden.

Cloninger, C. 1995. *Postcards for People Who Hurt*. Dallas: Word.

Hull, J. M. 1990. *Touching the Rock: An Experience of Blindness*. New York: Pantheon Books.

Kals, C. and J. F. Lauerman. 2000. "Fading of the Light." *Newsweek*, May 22, 78, 81.

Kear, N. C. 2014. *Now I See You*. Blackstone Audio.

Kübler-Ross, E. 1969. *On Death and Dying*. New York: The Macmillan Company.

Lucado, M. 2013. *You'll Get Through This*. Nashville: Thomas Nelson.

Rothschild, J. 2002. *Lessons I Learned in the Dark: Steps to Walking by Faith, Not by Sight*. Colorado Springs: Multnomah Books.

Yoken, C. 1979. *Living with Deaf Blindness: Nine Profiles*. Washington, D. C.: Gallaudet.

Chapter Three: History of Vision Theory and Biology of the Retina

Fitzgerald, B.A. 2018. "Using Hawkeye from the Avengers to communicate on the eye." *Advances In Physiology Education*, 42, no. 1: 90-98. https://journals.physiology.org/doi/full/10.1152/advan.00161.2017.

Kolb, H. 2003. "How the Retina Works." *American Scientist* 91: 28-35.

Lamb, T. D. 2001. "Evolution of the eye." *Scientific American*, July, 64-69.

Smith, A. M. 2015. *From Sight to Light: The Passage from Ancient to Modern Optics*. Chicago: University of Chicago.

Chapter Four: Eye Doctors, Eye Exams and Patient Advocacy
Haigh, D. 2018. 2020 On-site Blog; "How Your Eyes Change with Age," blog entry. May 10.

Wang, M. 2016. *From Darkness to Sight*. Nashville: Dunham.

Chapter Five: Symptoms of Macular Degeneration
The Angiogenesis Foundation, 2017, "Improving Long-Term Patient Outcomes for Exudative Age-Related Macular Degeneration." Version 1.0, 1-22.

AREDS Research Group, AREDS Report No. 8, 2001, "A Randomized, Placebo-Controlled, Clinical Trial of High-Dose Supplementation with Vitamins C and E, Beta Carotene, and Zinc for Age-Related Macular Degeneration and Vision Loss." Archives of Ophthalmology. 119:1417-1436.

Geller, A.M., P. A. Sieving and D. G. Green. 1992. "Effect on grating identification of sampling with degenerate arrays." *Journal of the Optical Society of America* 9: 472-477.

Geller, A. M. and P. A. Sieving. 1993. "Assessment of Foveal Cone Photoreceptors in Stargardt's Macular Dystrophy Using a Small Dot Detection Task." *Vision Research* 33: 1509-1524.

Sacks, O. 2009. "What hallucination reveals about our minds." TED talk. February. www.ted.com.

Chapter Six: Low Vision and Assistive Devices
Freeman, P. B. and R. T. Jose. 1991. *The Art and Practice of Low Vision*. Boston: Butterworth-Heinemann.

Ginsburg, A. P. 1983. "Contrast Sensitivity: Relating Visual Capability to Performance." *USAF Medical Service Digest*, Summer: 13-19.

Judith A. Read Low Vision Services. 2018. A program of United Disability Services. Akron, Ohio. Brochure.

Kals, C. and J. F. Lauerman. 2000. "Fading of the Light." *Newsweek*, May 22, 78, 81.

Chapter Seven: Daily Living
Better Vision. Better Life. 2010. n.d. Ridgefield, Connecticut: Eschenbach Optik of America. Brochure.

Freeman, P. B. and R. T. Jose. 1991. *The Art and Practice of Low*

Vision. Boston: Butterworth-Heinemann.

Grunwald, H. 1999. *Twilight: Losing Sight, Gaining Insight*. New York: Alfred A. Knopf.

Hull, J. M. 1990. *Touching the Rock: An Experience of Blindness*, New York: Pantheon Books.

Mogk, L. E. and M. Mogk. 2003. *Macular Degeneration: The Complete Guide to Saving and Maximizing Your Sight*. 2nd ed. New York: Ballantine.

Chapter Eight: Fifteen Again

Kleege, G. 1999. *Sight Unseen*. New Haven, Connecticut: Yale University.

Rothschild, J. 2002. *Lessons I Learned in the Dark: Steps to Walking by Faith, Not by Sight*. Colorado Springs: Multnomah Books.

Chapter Nine: The Lows of Public Transportation

Knighton, R. 2006. *Cockeyed: A Memoir*. New York: Public Affairs.

Chapter Ten: Adjustments in Social Life

Hull, J. M. 1990. *Touching the Rock: An Experience of Blindness*, New York: Pantheon Books.

Kals, C. and J. F. Lauerman. 2000. "Fading of the Light." *Newsweek*, May 22, 78, 81.

Kleege, G. 2015, Blind Creations.

Rothschild, J. 2002. *Lessons I Learned in the Dark: Steps to Walking by Faith, Not by Sight*. Colorado Springs: Multnomah Books.

Chapter Eleven: Employment Issues and Adjustments

Frederick, A. 2017. Blind Academics listserv. May 13.

Hull, J. M. 1990. *Touching the Rock: An Experience of Blindness*. New York: Pantheon Books.

Kleege, G. 1999. *Sight Unseen*. New Haven, Connecticut: Yale University.

Chapter Twelve: The Saga of Obtaining a Bioptic Driver's License

Chun, R., M. Cucuras and W. M. Jay. 2016. "Current perspectives of bioptic driving in low vision." *Neuroophthalmology* 40: 53-58.

Ginsburg, A. P. 1983. "Contrast sensitivity: Relating Visual Capability to Performance." *USAF Medical Service Digest*, Summer: 13-19.

The Northern Ohio Bioptic Driving Program. 2018. A program of United Disability Services. Akron, Ohio. Brochure.

Opportunities for Ohioans with Disabilities. 2018. Brochure.

Chapter Thirteen: Disability and the Blind Community

Cohen, L. H. 1994. *Train Go Sorry*. New York: Vintage.

Downey, C. 2013. "Design with the blind in mind." TED talk. October. www.ted.com.

Frederick, A. 2016. Blind Academics listserv. April 23.

Hull, J. M. 1990. *Touching the Rock: An Experience of Blindness*. New York: Pantheon Books.

Invisible Disabilities Association. https://invisibledisabilities.org/.

Johnson, A. 2006. *Privilege, Power, and Difference*, 2nd ed. New York: McGraw-Hill.

Kleege, G. 1999. *Sight Unseen*. New Haven, Connecticut: Yale University.

Rothschild, J. 2002. *Lessons I Learned in the Dark: Steps to Walking by Faith, Not by Sight*. Colorado Springs: Multnomah Books.

U.S. Census data. 2014. U.S. Department of Commerce, Economic & Statistics Administration, U.S. Census Bureau. www.census.gov.

Acknowledgments

Bolte Taylor, J. 2006. *My Stroke of Insight: A Brain Scientist's Personal Journey*. Large print ed. Detroit: Gale Cengage Learning.

Deaver, M. K. 2001. *A Different Drummer: My Thirty Years with Ronald Reagan*. Large print ed. New York: Harper.

Fox, M. J. 2002. *Lucky Man*. New York: Random House.

Runyan, M. 2001. *No Finish Line: My Life as I See It*. New York: G.P. Putnam Sons.

Lightning Source UK Ltd.
Milton Keynes UK
UKHW020648170223
417189UK00015B/487